Renal diet cookbook 2021

- Quick, Easy, and Flavorful Recipes for Every Stage of Kidney Disease -

[Simona Malcom]

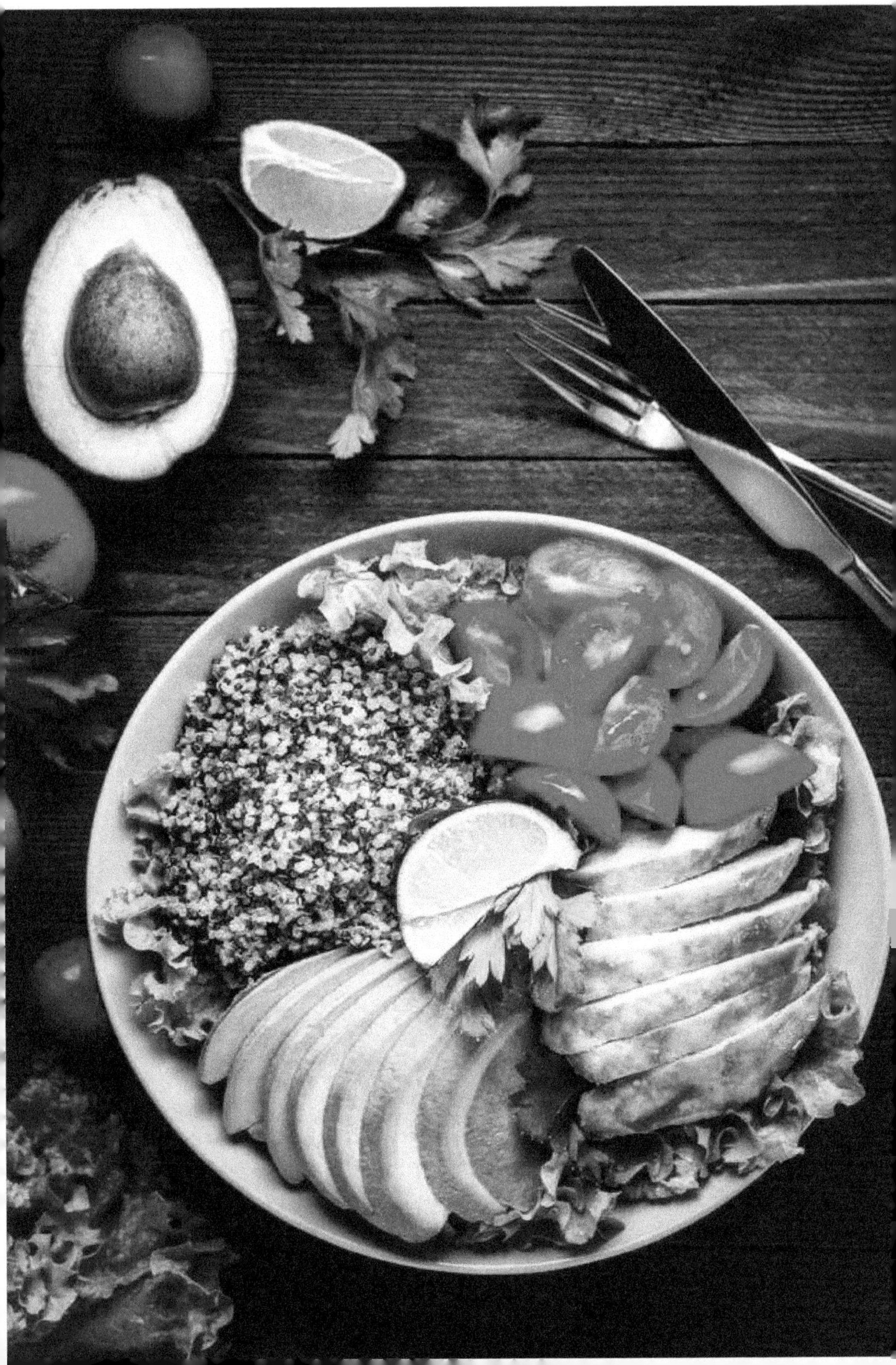

Table Of Contents

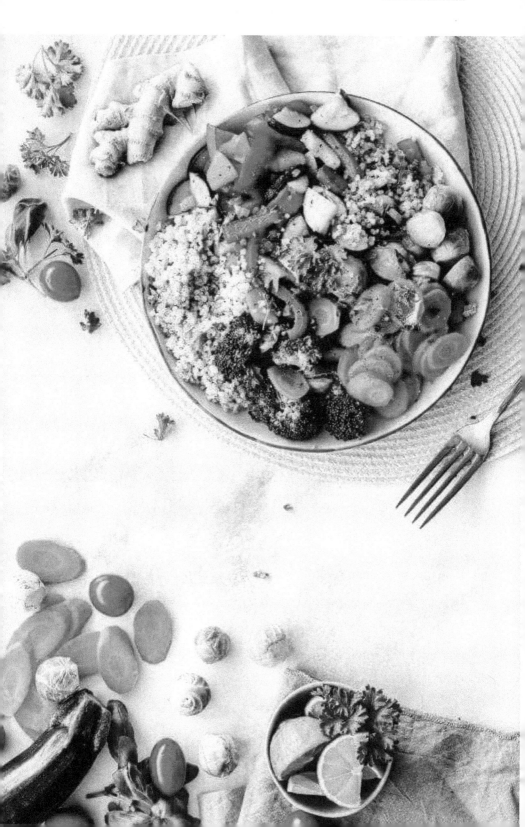

The following Book is reproduced below with the goal of providing information that is as accurate and reliable as possible. Regardless, purchasing this Book can be seen as consent to the fact that both the publisher and the author of this book are in no way experts on the topics discussed within and that any recommendations or suggestions that are made herein are for entertainment purposes only. Professionals should be consulted as needed prior to undertaking any of the action endorsed herein.

This declaration is deemed fair and valid by both the American Bar Association and the Committee of Publishers Association and is legally binding throughout the United States.

Furthermore, the transmission, duplication, or reproduction of any of the following work including specific information will be considered an illegal act irrespective of if it is done electronically or in print. This extends to creating a secondary or tertiary copy of the work or a recorded copy and is only allowed with the express written consent from the Publisher. All additional right reserved.

The information in the following pages is broadly considered a truthful and accurate account of facts and as such, any inattention, use, or misuse of the information in question by the reader will render any resulting actions solely under their purview. There are no scenarios in which the publisher or the original author of this work can be in any fashion deemed liable for any hardship or damages that may befall them after undertaking information described herein.

Additionally, the information in the following pages is intended only for informational purposes and should thus be thought of as universal. As befitting its nature, it is presented without assurance regarding its prolonged validity or interim quality. Trademarks that are mentioned are done without written consent and can in no way be considered an endorsement from the trademark holder.

Introduction

Human health hangs in a complete balance when all of its interconnected bodily mechanisms function properly in perfect sync. Without its major organs working normally, the body soon suffers indelible damage. Kidney malfunction is one such example, and it is not just the entire water balance that is disturbed by the kidney disease, but a number of other diseases also emerge due to this problem.

Kidney diseases are progressive, meaning that they can ultimately lead to permanent kidney damage if left unchecked and uncontrolled. That is why it is essential to control and manage the disease and halt its progress, which can be done through medicinal and natural means. While medicines can guarantee only thirty percent of the cure, a change of lifestyle and diet can prove miraculous with their seventy percent guaranteed results. A kidney-friendly diet and lifestyle not only saves the kidneys from excess minerals, but it also aids medicines to work actively. Treatment without a good diet, hence, proves to be useless. In this renal diet cookbook, we shall bring out the basic facts about kidney diseases, their symptoms, causes, and diagnosis. This preliminary introduction can help the readers understand the problem clearly; then, we shall discuss the role of renal diet and kidney-friendly lifestyle in curbing the diseases. It's not just that the book also contains a range of delicious renal diet recipes, which will guarantee luscious flavors and good health.

Despite their tiny size, the kidneys perform a number of functions, which are vital for the body to be able to function healthily.

These include:

- Filtering excess fluids and waste from the blood.

- Creating the enzyme known as renin, which regulates blood pressure.

- Ensuring bone marrow creates red blood cells.

- Controlling calcium and phosphorus levels through absorption and excretion.

Unfortunately, when kidney disease reaches a chronic stage, these functions start to stop working. However, with the right treatment and lifestyle, it is possible to manage symptoms and continue living well. This is even more applicable in the earlier stages of the disease. Tactlessly, 10% of all adults over the age of 20 will experience some form of kidney disease in their lifetime. There are a variety of different treatments for kidney disease, which depend on the cause of the disease.

According to international stats, kidney (or renal) diseases are affecting around 14% of the adult population. In the US, approx. 661.000 Americans suffer from kidney dysfunction. Out of these patients, 468.000 proceed to dialysis treatment, and the rest have one active kidney transplant.

The high quantities of diabetes and heart illness are also related to kidney dysfunction, and sometimes one condition, for example, diabetes, may prompt the other.

With such a significant number of high rates, possibly the best course of treatment is the contravention of dialysis, making people depend upon clinical and crisis facility meds in any occasion multiple times every week. In this manner, if your kidney has just given a few indications of brokenness, you can forestall dialysis through an eating routine, something that we will talk about in this book.

CHAPTER 1: **BREAKFAST**

Salmon Bagel

Prep:5 mins
Cook:5 mins
Servings:1

Ingredients

1 slice whole-grain bread toasted
1 ½ ounces sliced smoked salmon
2 tablespoons reduced-fat cream cheese softened
1/4 teaspoon everything bagel seasoning

Directions

1

Top toast with cream cheese, salmon and seasoning.

Nutrition

Serving Size: 1 Slice

:

181 calories; protein 13.7g; carbohydrates 13.9g; dietary fiber 2g; sugars 3.4g; fat 7.6g; saturated fat 3.4g; cholesterol 26mg; vitamin a iu 202.9IU; vitamin c 0.1mg; folate 26.4mcg; calcium 79.3mg; iron 1.1mg; magnesium 31.4mg; potassium 212.7mg; sodium 589.6mg.

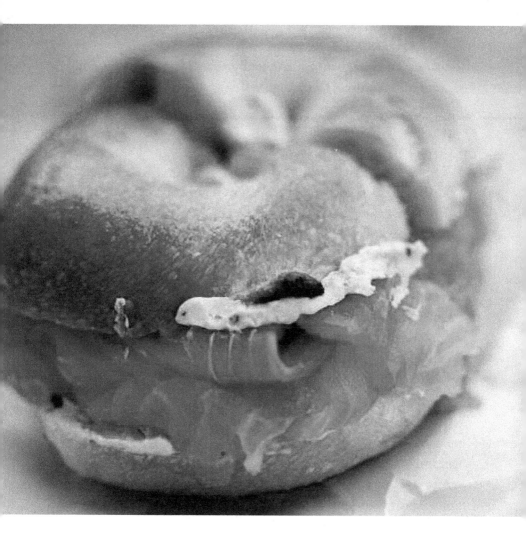

TEX-MEX OMELET

Prep: 5 mins
Cook: 10 mins
Servings: 4

INGREDIENTS

Roasted Cherry Tomato Salsa (quantities below yield enough for 1 saucy to 2 not-so-saucy omelets)
½ pint cherry tomatoes
1/4 small white onion chopped
1 cloves garlic minced
⅓ cup loosely packed cilantro chopped
1/2 jalapeño, deseeded and membranes removed, finely chopped
1 teaspoons white wine vinegar
1/4 teaspoon olive oil
⅛ teaspoon sea salt
Tex-Mex Omelet (quantities below yield 1 omelet)
2 eggs
2 tablespoons milk or water
pinch black pepper
3 tablespoons black beans
hot sauce (Cholula recommended)
1 scant tablespoon butter
⅓ cup Jack cheese or other melty cheese, shredded
pinch sea salt
handful blue corn chips or tortilla chips, broken into small bite-sized pieces
optional garnishes: sliced avocado, sour cream, hot sauce, etc.

DIRECTIONS

Make the salsa: Preheat the oven to 400 degrees Fahrenheit. Line a small, rimmed baking pan with parchment paper for easy clean-up. Toss the cherry tomatoes with ½ teaspoon olive oil and a sprinkle of sea salt on the baking pan. Roast for 17 to 20 minutes, until the tomatoes are juicy and collapsing on themselves.

In a bowl, mix together the chopped onion, cilantro, jalapeño, garlic, vinegar and sea salt. Once the tomatoes have cooled enough to handle, use a serrated knife to chop them. Pull off the tomato skins as you go for a smoother salsa. Mix the tomatoes into the mixture. Taste and add more salt or lime juice if necessary.

Make the omelet: In a bowl, whisk together the eggs, milk or water, sea salt, black pepper and a few dashes of hot sauce. You want the egg mixture to be super scrambled. Heat an 8-inch, well-seasoned cast iron skillet or non-stick skillet over medium-low heat. Once the pan is hot that a drop of water sizzles on contact, toss in the pat of butter and swirl the pan to coat. Pour in the egg mixture and let it set for about 15 seconds. Use a heat-safe spatula to gently scoot the set eggs toward the middle of the pan, then tilt the pan so runny eggs take their place. Repeat this process until there is hardly any runny eggs to scoot around. Use your spatula to gently release the underside of the omelet from the pan. Tilt the pan a little forward and back to make sure it's not stuck anywhere, then use a quick flick of the wrist to flip the omelet back into the pan. Let it set for a few seconds, then scoot it off the pan onto a plate.

Immediately top ½ of the warm omelet with a sprinkle of cheese, followed by black beans, smashed tortilla chips, and more cheese, then gently fold the other half on top. Spoon a generous amount of salsa (warm the salsa first if necessary) over the middle of the omelet as shown. Serve immediately.

Nutritions:

Total fat 37g

Cholesterol 447.5mg

Sogium 1960.9mg

Vegetable Rice Casserole

Prep: 15 minutes
Cook: minutes
Servings: 10

Ingredients

3 cups of dry/UNCOOKED instant brown rice, cooked according to package.
1 (10 oz) bag of frozen broccoli
3 1/2 cups peeled and diced carrots
2 (10.5 oz each) containers of organic cream of mushroom soup
2 medium onions, diced
8 large cloves of garlic, minced
1 (10 oz) bag of frozen peas
3/4 cup fresh parsley, chopped
1 teaspoon cracked black pepper
2 1/2 cups parmesan cheese, freshly grated
2 cups sharp cheddar cheese, freshly grated
2 tablespoons olive oil
1 teaspoon sea salt

DIRECTIONS

Measure 3 cups of dry instant rice and cook according to package

Combine onion, garlic, carrots, olive oil, salt, and pepper in a large skillet

Sautee for 15 minutes on medium high heat, until carrots start to soften and onions become translucent

Add peas, mushroom soup, broccoli, 1 1/2 cups parmesan cheese, and 1 cup of sharp cheddar cheese to the skillet

Stir on medium heat until heated through, about 10 - 15 minutes

Add cooked rice and parsley to skillet and stir to combine

Transfer mixture to a 13 x 9 casserole dish

Top with remaining 1 cup of parmesan cheese and 1 cup of sharp cheddar cheese

Bake for 10-12 minutes at 400 degrees, until cheese is bubbly and beginning to brown

Nutrition

Calories 415
Total fat 26g
Cholesterol 66mg
Fiber 3g
Sodium 1000mg
Carbs 25g
Protein 21g

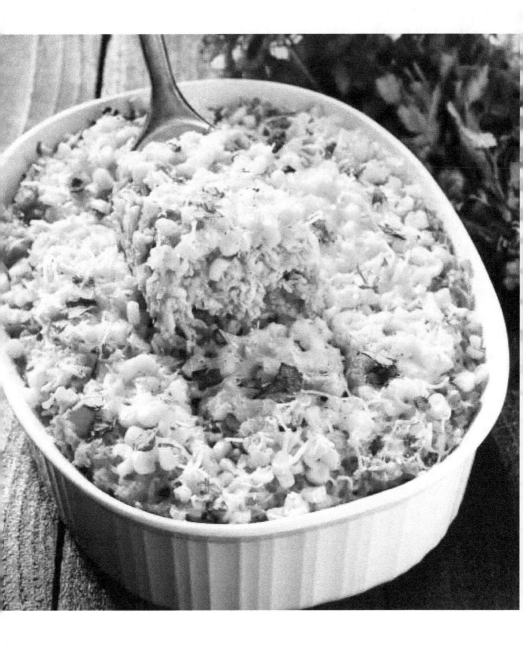

Healthy Melon Shake

Prep: 7 mins
Cook: 0 mins
Servings. 1

Ingredients

Hami Melon or Tuscan Style Cantaloupe
Lime juice
Greek yogurt (Vanilla or Plain)
Bananas, frozen
Galia melon
Milk

Directions

Gather all of your Ingredients and slice the melon into cubes.
Place all Ingredients into your blender, and blend until smooth.
Make adjustments as needed if you'd like it thicker or thinner!

Mushroom and Tofu Scramble

Prep Time: 20 minutes
Cook Time: 15 minutes
Servings: 3

Ingredients

1 lb firm or extra firm tofu (drained and pressed)
1 ½ cups mushrooms (sliced)
¼ of an onion (diced)
2 tsp dried parsley
½ cup halved cherry tomatoes
1 garlic clove (minced)
½ tsp smoked paprika
½ teaspoon dry mustard
¼ teaspoon tumeric
¼ teaspoon cumin
½ teaspoon salt
⅛ teaspoon pepper

Directions

Drain your tofu and press it for at least 20 minutes.
Wrap your block of tofu in a paper towel and put it on a plate.
Put another plate over the top and weigh it down with bags of dried beans.
In a skillet over medium heat, sauté onion and garlic in 1 tbsp water for a few minutes until soft.
Add the mushrooms and saute until they reduce in volume.
Crumble the tofu into the skillet, add spices and stir to combine.
Cook for a few more minutes to heat through and let the flavors meld.
Take off heat, add tomatoes, stir again to combine.
Serve hot.

Mediterranean Easy Toast

Prep: 5 mins
Cook: 5 Mins
Servings: 1

INGREDIENTS

4 thick slices whole grain or whole wheat bread of choice
½ cup/123 g hummus
1 cucumber, sliced into rounds
2 tbsp/about 16 g chopped olives of your choice
Za'atar spice blend, to your liking
Handful baby arugula
Crumbled feta cheese, a sprinkle to your liking
1 to 2 Roma tomatoes, sliced into rounds

DIRECTIONS

Toast bread slices to your liking
Spread about 2 tbsp hummus on each slice of bread.
Add a generous sprinkle of Za'atar spice,
then load on the arugula and remaining toppings.

Egg Whites Cups

Prep: 5 Mins
Cook: 5 Mins
Servings: 4

Ingredients

for 6 servings
1 roma tomato, 11 calories
2 cups egg white(480 mL), 250 calories
1 roma tomato, 11 calories
salt, to taste, 0 calories
2 cups spinach(60 g), 14 calories
½ teaspoon pepper, 0 calories

Directions

Preheat the oven to 350°F.
Lightly grease a muffin tin.
Then divide equally the spinach across 6 cups.
Dice the tomato, then fill the cups with the tomato and egg whites.
Season with salt and pepper.
Bake for 15 minutes, or until the whites have set.
Serve hot.
Enjoy!

Nutritions:

Fat 9g
Carbs 1g
Fiber 0g
Sugar 0g
Protein 12g

ROSEMARY FRITTATA

Prep: 5 mins
Cook: 10 mins
Servings: 2

Ingredients

8 pastured eggs
1 tablespoons fresh rosemary minced
1/4 teaspoon sea salt
Pinch red pepper flakes
2 cups of finely chopped greens such as mustard, collards, kale, chard
1/4 teaspoon black pepper
4 tablespoons butter
1/2 medium-sized onion minced
1/2 cup shredded Parmesan cheese
2 tablespoons sun-dried tomatoes minced (optional)

Directions

Preheat oven grill to high. Spray a medium ovenproof pan with oil and set over a medium heat. Add red onion and cook, stirring, for 10 minutes, until softened. Add courgette and cook for 2 minutes. Add rosemary and potato slices and cook, gently stirring, until potatoes are browned.

Spread vegetable mixture evenly in pan. In a small bowl, combine eggs and milk. Pour egg mixture over vegetables, tilting the pan to spread egg mixture evenly. Add rocket. Cook for 2-3 minutes, until bottom of frittata is set.

Sprinkle frittata with cheese. Place under grill and cook for 2-3 minutes, until cheese is golden.

Divide frittata between two plates. Season with black pepper and serve with salad drizzled in vinaigrette and chutney on side.

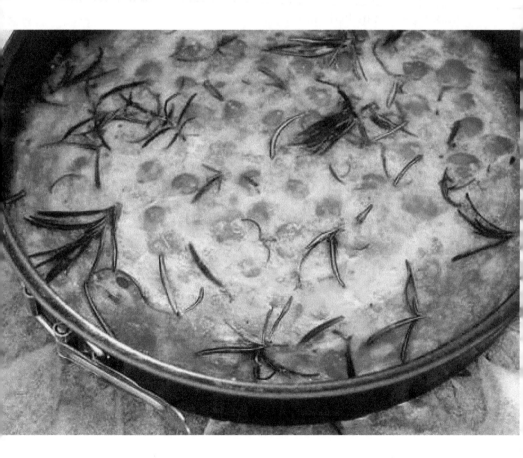

Classic French Crepes

Prep:5 mins
Cook:30 mins
Servings:12

Directions:

Sift together flour, sugar and salt; set aside. In a large bowl, beat eggs and milk together with an electric mixer. Beat in flour mixture until smooth; stir in melted butter.

Heat a lightly oiled griddle or frying pan over medium high heat. Pour or scoop the batter onto the griddle, using 2 tablespoons for each crepe. Tip and rotate pan to spread batter as thinly as possible. Brown on both sides and serve hot.

Nutritions

94 calories
protein 4g
carbohydrates 10.3g
fat 4.1g
cholesterol 54.8mg
sodium 96.5mg.

Exotic Juice

Prep:15 mins
Servings:12

Ingredients

1 seedless watermelon, halved and sliced
3 cups water
lime, juiced
1 (15.25 ounce) can crushed pineapple
½ cup shredded coconut
1 (12 fluid ounce) can evaporated milk
2 tablespoons white sugar, or to taste (Optional)

Directions

Grate watermelon with a fork from the rind into a large bowl, leaving
no large chunks. Stir water, pineapple, evaporated milk, and coconut
into the grated watermelon. Add sugar; stir until dissolved. Squeeze
lime juice into the watermelon mixture.

Nutrition

200 calories;
protein 4.7g;
carbohydrates 41.1g;
fat 3.8g;
cholesterol 9.1mg;
sodium 48.1mg.

Berry Frozen Yogurt

Prep:15 mins
Cook:2 hrs
Servings:4

Ingredients

3 cups plain low-fat yogurt
2 cups blueberries, raspberries and sliced strawberries, mixed
1 cup blueberries, raspberries and sliced strawberries, mixed
1 (1.5 ounce) envelope instant sugar-free vanilla pudding mix
1 tablespoon white sugar
1 tablespoon fresh lemon juice
¾ cup wheat and barley nugget cereal

Directions

Combine the yogurt and pudding mix in a large bowl; beat with an electric mixer until well blended, 1 to 2 minutes. Stir in 2 cups of the mixed berries and the cereal until blended. Pour the yogurt and berry mixture into a 9 inch pie plate. Cover with plastic wrap, and refrigerate 2 hours.

Meanwhile, place the remaining 1 cup of berries in a medium bowl and slightly mash with a fork. Stir in the sugar and lemon juice. Set mixture aside at room temperature.

Nutrition

406 calories
protein 13.5g
carbohydrates 58.7g
fat 14.7g
cholesterol 51.8mg
sodium 708.8mg.

Coconut Flour Pancakes

Prep:15 mins
Cook:15 mins
Servings:6

Ingredients

1 ½ cups coconut flour
½ teaspoon salt
½ cup rice flour
2 teaspoons baking powder
1 teaspoon baking soda
3 cups buttermilk
5 eggs, separated
¼ cup butter, melted
2 teaspoons macadamia nut oil, or more as needed
1 teaspoon almond extract

Directions

Whisk coconut flour, rice flour, baking powder, baking soda, and salt together in a bowl. Mix buttermilk, egg yolks, butter, and almond extract together in a separate bowl.

Heat griddle to 350 degrees F or a skillet over medium-high heat; lightly grease with macadamia nut oil.

Beat egg whites in a glass or metal bowl until medium peaks form. Lift your beater or whisk straight up: the tip of the peak formed by the egg whites should curl over slightly.

Stir buttermilk mixture into flour mixture; fold in egg whites, 1/3 at a time, until batter is just mixed and thick.

Ladle batter onto the griddle and cook until bubbles form and the edges are dry, 3 to 4 minutes. Flip and cook until browned on the other side, 2 to 3 minutes. Repeat with remaining batter.

Nutrition

240 calories
protein 10.2g;
carbohydrates 17.2g
fat 14.6g
cholesterol 180.2mg
sodium 807.5mg.

Delicious Rice Milk Waffles

Prep:15 mins
Cook:5 mins
Servings:4

Ingredients

2 eggs, separated
1 ¾ cups rice milk
1 tablespoon white sugar
¾ cup modified tapioca starch
½ cup canola oil
1 cup rice flour
2 teaspoons baking powder
½ teaspoon vanilla extract
¼ cup almond meal
¼ teaspoon salt
cooking spray

Directions

Preheat a waffle iron according to manufacturer's DIRECTIONS.
Beat egg whites in a glass, metal, or ceramic bowl with an electric
mixer until stiff peaks form.

Mix egg yolks in a separate bowl using a hand beater. Beat in rice milk,
rice flour, tapioca starch, oil, almond meal, sugar, baking powder,
vanilla extract, and salt just until smooth. Fold in stiff egg whites.
Spray the preheated waffle iron with cooking spray. Cook waffles until
golden brown and the iron stops steaming, about 5 minutes per waffle.

:

Nutrition

623 calories

protein 9.8g

carbohydrates 71.6g

fat 33.4g

cholesterol 93mg

sodium 463.2mg

Chinese Stir – Fried Tomatoes Eggs

Prep:10 mins
Cook:5 mins
Servings:3

Ingredients

6 eggs, beaten
2 green onions, thinly sliced
4 ripe tomatoes, sliced into wedges
2 tablespoons avocado oil

Directions

Heat 1 tablespoon avocado oil in a wok or skillet over medium heat. Cook and stir eggs in the hot oil until mostly cooked through, 1 minute. Transfer eggs to a plate.

Pour remaining 1 tablespoon avocado oil into wok; cook and stir tomatoes until liquid has mostly evaporated, about 3 minutes. Return eggs to wok and add green onions; cook and stir until eggs are fully cooked, about 30 seconds.

Nutrition

:

264 calories
protein 14.5g
carbohydrates 9.2g
fat 19.7g
cholesterol 372mg
sodium 151.5mg

Rice Milk Pancakes

Prep:10 mins
Cook:20 mins
Servings:4

Ingredients

1 cup sweet rice flour
2 tablespoons vegetable oil
½ teaspoon salt
2 eggs, beaten
1¼ cups soy yogurt
1 teaspoon baking soda
1 teaspoons baking powder
¼ cup rice milk

Directions

Sift the rice flour, baking powder, baking soda, cinnamon, and salt in a bowl. In another bowl, whisk together the beaten eggs, soy yogurt, rice milk, and oil, and pour into the flour mixture. Stir briefly just to combine.

Heat a lightly oiled griddle or frying pan over medium-high heat. Scoop about 1/4 cup of batter per pancake onto the heated griddle, and cook for 2 minutes, until bubbles appear on the surface. Flip the pancake and cook 2 minutes more, until the pancake is golden brown on both sides.

Nutrition

310 calories;
protein 9.8g;

carbohydrates 37.7g;
fat 13.4g;
cholesterol 93mg;
sodium 737.9mg.

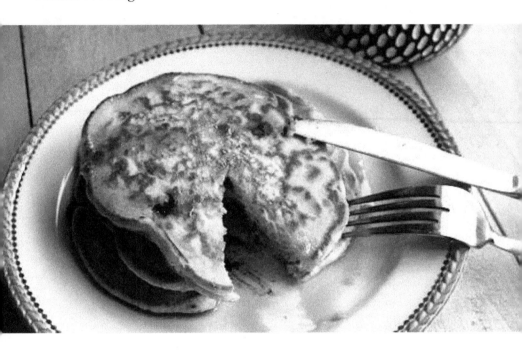

Crispy Chicken Egg Rolls

Prep:30 mins
Cook:15 mins
Servings:14

Ingredients

½ pound cooked chicken breast
⅓ cup diced celery
1 egg
2 ounces cream cheese
1 tablespoon Louisiana-style hot sauce
2 ounces blue cheese
salt
freshly ground black pepper
14 wonton wrappers, or more as needed
cayenne pepper
1 tablespoon water
oil for frying

Directions

Dice chicken into small cubes. Transfer to a mixing bowl. Add celery, blue cheese, cream cheese, and hot sauce. Season with salt, black pepper, and cayenne pepper. Mix with a spoon until filling is well combined.

2

Beat egg and water together. Brush egg wash over the edges of 1 wonton wrapper. Place a heaping tablespoon of filling near one edge. Spread out with your fingers, leaving a 1/2-inch border. Roll edge up over filling. Crimp in both edges and roll over once more. Fold in about 1/4 inch of dough on either side to seal the ends. Apply more egg wash on top and continue rolling. Place on a plastic-lined baking pan. Repeat with remaining wonton wrappers and filling.

3

Fill a skillet with enough oil to reach halfway up the egg rolls. Heat to 350 degrees F in a skillet over medium heat. Add a batch of egg rolls; fry until browned and crispy, 2 minutes per side. Drain on a paper towel-lined plate. Fry remaining egg rolls.

Nutrition

121 calories
protein 6.4g
carbohydrates 5g
fat 8.2g
cholesterol 34.1mg
sodium 169.9mg.

Cinnamon French Toast Strata

Prep:20 mins
Cook:1 hr 30 mins
Additional:13 hrs 10 mins
Servings:15

Ingredients

¾ cup butter, melted
1 teaspoon ground cinnamon
2 (21 ounce) cans apple pie filling
20 slices white bread
6 eggs
1 cup brown sugar
1 ½ cups milk
½ cup maple syrup
1 teaspoon vanilla extract

Directions

Grease a 9x13 inch baking pan. In a small bowl, stir together the melted butter, brown sugar and cinnamon.
    2
Spread the sugar mixture into the bottom of the prepared pan. Spread the apple pie filling evenly over the sugar mixture. Layer the bread slices on top of the filling, pressing down as you go. In a medium bowl, beat the eggs with the milk and vanilla. Slowly pour this mixture over the bread, making sure that it is completely absorbed. Cover the pan with aluminum foil and refrigerate overnight.
    3
In the morning, preheat oven to 350 degrees F.
    4

Place covered pan into the oven and bake at 350 degrees F for 60 to 75 minutes. When done remove from oven and turn on broiler. Remove foil and drizzle maple syrup on top of the egg topping; broil for 2 minutes, or until the syrup begins to caramelize. Remove from the oven and let stand for 10 minutes, then cut into squares. Invert the pan onto a serving tray or baking sheet so the apple filling is on top. Serve hot.

Nutrition

375 calories;
protein 6.1g
carbohydrates 60.5g
fat 12.9g
cholesterol 100.8mg
sodium 370.4mg.

Savoury Buckwheat Granola

Prep:10 mins
Cook:40 mins
Additional:1 hr
Servings:10

Ingredients

2 cups rolled oats
¾ cup buckwheat groats, chopped
1 pinch salt
3 tablespoons coconut oil
¼ cup honey
1 vanilla bean, split and scraped
¾ cup sunflower seeds
½ cup sweetened flaked coconut
½ cup raisins
½ cup almonds, chopped

Directions

oven to 300 degrees F . Line a baking sheet with parchment paper.
    2
Mix oats, buckwheat, sunflower seeds, and salt in a large bowl.
    3
Melt coconut oil in a small saucepan over medium heat; stir in honey
and seeds from vanilla bean until mixed. Pour over oat mixture and
toss to coat. Spread oat mixture evenly over prepared baking sheet.
    4
Bake in the preheated oven, stirring every 10 minutes, until granola is
lightly brown, 35 to 40 minutes. Stir almonds into granola and
continue baking until golden grown, about 5 to 10 minutes more.

Allow granola to cool completely, then stir in coconut and raisins. Store in an airtight container.

Nutrition

304 calories
protein 7.5g
carbohydrates 40g
fat 14.6g
sodium 13.9mg.

Apple Muesli

Prep:10 mins
Cook:20 mins
Servings:4

Ingredients

¾ cup water
½ teaspoon ground cinnamon
¼ cup white sugar
4 apples - peeled, cored and chopped

Directions

In a saucepan, combine apples, water, sugar, and cinnamon. Cover, and cook over medium heat for 18 minutes, or until apples are soft. Allow to cool, then mash with a fork or potato masher.

Nutrition

121 calories;
protein 0.4g;
carbohydrates 31.8g;
fat 0.2g;
sodium 2.7mg

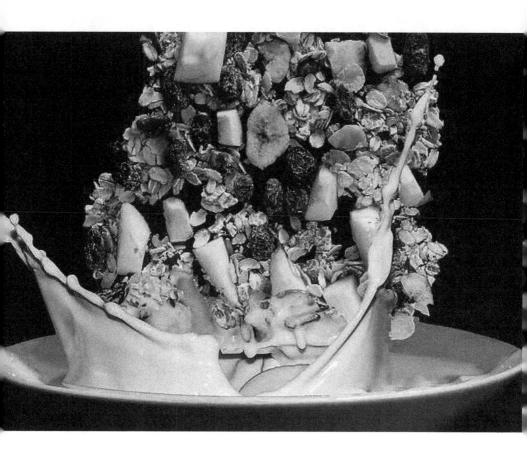

Sun Dried Tomato Frittata

Prep:20 mins
Cook:20 mins
Additional:5 mins
Servings:12

Ingredients

Cooking spray
12 large eggs
5 slices Fully Cooked Bacon
¼ teaspoon freshly ground black pepper
1 cup cherry tomatoes, quartered
½ cup fresh baby arugula leaves, chopped
½ cup shredded Cheddar cheese
½ teaspoon kosher salt
½ cup green onions, finely sliced
½ teaspoon hot sauce

Directions

Preheat oven to 350 degrees F and spray a 12-cup muffin tin lightly
with cooking spray.
  2
Crumble Smithfield® fully cooked bacon into small pieces and place
into a small bowl.
  3
Place eggs into a large mixing bowl. Whisk until combined. Add
bacon, tomatoes, arugula, cheese, green onions, salt, hot sauce, and
pepper. Whisk gently until Ingredients are combined.
  4

Use a 1/3 cup to pour egg mixture into prepared muffin cups. Bake for 25 minutes, or until eggs are set. Remove and let sit for 3 to 5 minutes before transferring to serving plates. Serve warm.

Nutrition

103 calories
protein 8.1g
carbohydrates 1.4g
fat 7.3g
cholesterol 193mg
sodium 217mg.

MEXICAN BREAKFAST FRITTATA

Prep:15 mins
Cook:35 mins
Servings:2

Ingredients

cooking spray
4 egg whites
1 red bell pepper, cut into thin strips
1 medium white onion, thinly sliced
¼ cup milk
1 pinch ground cumin
1 teaspoon olive oil
2 eggs
½ teaspoon salt
½ teaspoon ground black pepper
½ cup salsa

Directions

Preheat the oven to 350 degrees F. Spray a small casserole dish with cooking spray.

Heat oil in a 12-inch nonstick skillet over medium heat. Add bell pepper and onion and cook until tender, about 5 minutes.

While pepper and onion are cooking, combine milk, egg whites, whole eggs, salt, pepper, and cumin into a medium bowl using a whisk.

Transfer cooked vegetables to the prepared casserole dish. Pour egg mixture over the top.

Bake in the preheated oven until eggs are set, about 30 minutes.

Remove frittata from the oven and cut into wedges or squares. Place onto a plate and top with salsa.

Nutrition

202 calories
protein 16.9g
carbohydrates 15.6g
fat 8.5g
cholesterol 188.4mg
sodium 1169mg.

Fresh Rhubarb Muffin

Prep:10 mins
Cook:25 mins
Servings:12

Ingredients

2 tablespoons butter, melted

¾ cup brown sugar

2 tablespoons vegetable oil

1 egg

1 ⅓ cups all-purpose flour

½ teaspoon baking soda

 cup vanilla yogurt

¼ teaspoon salt

1 cup diced rhubarb

¼ teaspoon ground nutmeg

 cup brown sugar

½ teaspoon ground cinnamon

¼ cup crushed sliced almonds

2 teaspoons melted butter

Directions

Preheat the oven to 350 degrees F. Grease a 12 cup muffin tin, or line with paper liners.

2

In a medium bowl, stir together the yogurt, 2 tablespoons of melted butter, oil and egg. In a large bowl, stir together the flour, 3/4 cup of brown sugar, baking soda and salt. Pour the wet Ingredients into the dry, and mix until just blended. Fold in rhubarb. Spoon into the prepared muffin tin, filling cups at least 2/3 full.

3

In a small bowl, stir together 1/4 cup of brown sugar, cinnamon, nutmeg, almonds, and 2 teaspoons of melted butter. Spoon over the tops of the muffins, and press down lightly.

4

Bake for 25 minutes in the preheated oven, or until the tops spring back when lightly pressed. Cool in the pan for 15 minutes before removing.

Nutrition

192 calories
protein 3g
carbohydrates 31g
fat 6.6g
cholesterol 22.9mg
sodium 137.7mg.

Roasted Pepper Soup

Prep: 10 mins
Cook: 25 mins
Servings:2

Ingredients

1 green bell pepper
1 large orange bell pepper
1 large red bell pepper
yellow bell pepper
¼ teaspoon garlic salt
8 cloves garlic
½ lemon
3 cups vegetable broth
¼ teaspoon dried thyme
ground black pepper to taste
1 teaspoon fennel seed

Directions

Preheat oven to 375 degrees F , halve all peppers and peel garlic.
   2
Place halved peppers, cut side up in shallow baking dish. Place one garlic clove in each half and squeeze lemon juice generously over peppers. Roast for 1 hour.
   3
Meanwhile pour vegetable broth into a 2 quart sauce pan and add fennel seeds. Bring to boil, cover and simmer.
   4
When peppers are done, remove from oven and set aside to cool. When cool enough to touch peel skin from peppers.
   5

Strain fennel seeds from broth and return to a boil. Add thyme and simmer 15 minutes, reducing amount of broth.

6

Slice a 1 inch section from each color of pepper and cut into pieces. Set aside for later garnishing.

7

In a blender, place remaining peppers, garlic and a 1/2 cup broth on blend just long enough to shred the peppers, but not puree them. You want to see the different colors. Pour the blended peppers into the broth and stir well. Add garlic salt and black pepper to taste, then add garnishing pepper pieces and enjoy.

Nutrition

157 calories
protein 5.9g
carbohydrates 33.8g
fat 1.8g
sodium 928.9mg.

Happy Millet Muffins

Prep:10 mins
Cook:15 mins
Servings:16

Ingredients

2 ¼ cups whole wheat flour
½ cup honey
1 cup buttermilk
⅓ cup millet
teaspoon baking powder
teaspoon salt
1 teaspoon baking soda
1 egg, lightly beaten
½ cup vegetable oil

Directions

Preheat oven to 400 degrees F (200 degrees C). Grease 16 muffin cups.

2

In a large bowl, mix the whole wheat flour, millet flour, baking powder, baking soda, and salt. In a separate bowl, mix the buttermilk, egg, vegetable oil, and honey. Stir buttermilk mixture into the flour mixture just until evenly moist. Transfer batter to the prepared muffin cups.

3

Bake 15 minutes in the preheated oven, or until a toothpick inserted in the center of a muffin comes out clean.

Nutrition

176 calories

protein 3.7g
carbohydrates 24.8g
fat 7.7g
cholesterol 12.2mg
sodium 268.4mg.

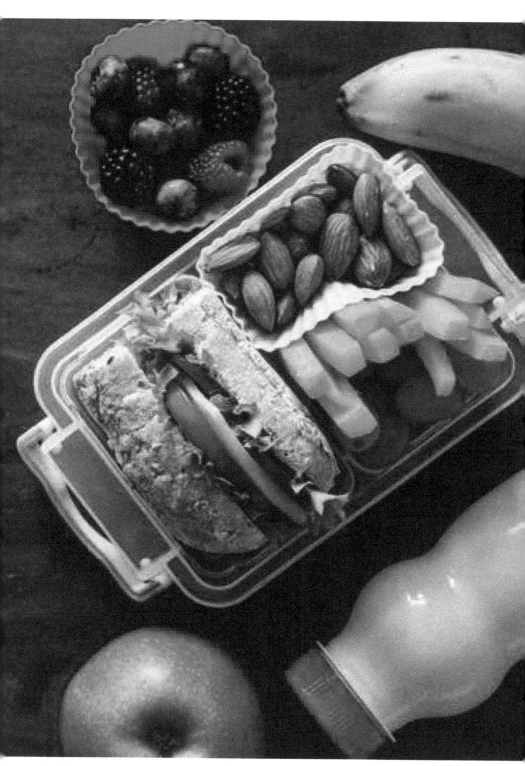

CHAPTER 2: LUNCH

Pasta with Chicken and Asparagus

Prep:20 mins
Cook:15 mins
Servings:8

Ingredients

⅓ cup corn oil
4 Roma tomatoes, chopped
4 skinless, boneless chicken breast halves, cubed
4 cloves garlic, minced
1 cup heavy whipping cream
4 Roma tomatoes, chopped
1 teaspoon salt
ground black pepper to taste
1 (16 ounce) package fresh linguini pasta
½ cup white wine
1 pound fresh asparagus, sliced
½ cup freshly grated Parmesan cheese

Directions

Heat corn oil in a skillet over medium heat. Cook and stir chicken and garlic until chicken is no longer pink in the center and juices run clear, 5 to 7 minutes. Transfer chicken to a plate.

2
Pour wine in the same skillet and simmer, about 2 minutes.

3
Stir cream into simmering wine; reduce heat and simmer until large bubbles appear, 3 to 4 minutes.

4

Cook and stir chicken, tomatoes, salt, and black pepper into cream mixture until all Ingredients are warmed, 2 minutes.

5

Bring a large pot of lightly salted water to a boil. Stir in pasta and asparagus; cook until pasta floats to the top, 3 minutes. Drain.

6

Toss pasta and asparagus together with chicken and cream sauce. Top with Parmesan cheese.

Nutrition

494 calories; protein 25.4g; carbohydrates 42g; fat 24g; cholesterol 125.6mg; sodium 431.1mg.

Sicilian Calamari Salad

Prep:15 mins
Cook:10 mins
Servings:8

Ingredients

½ cup olive oil
1 jalapeno pepper, finely chopped
¼ cup red wine vinegar
2 cloves garlic, pressed
1 cup water
1 pound squid, cleaned and cut into rings and tentacles
1 cup dry white wine
1 cup chopped celery
½ bunch chopped fresh cilantro
1 green bell pepper, chopped
1 yellow bell pepper, chopped
1 cup chopped cucumber
1 bunch fresh green onions, chopped
1 bunch chopped fresh parsley
1 red bell pepper, chopped
1 cup jicama, peeled and shredded

Directions

In a small bowl, mix the olive oil, red wine vinegar, and garlic.
   2
In a medium saucepan, bring the wine and water to a low boil. Stir in the squid and cook until opaque, about 2 minutes. Drain and cool.
   3
In a large bowl, mix the celery, cilantro, green bell pepper, red bell pepper, yellow bell pepper, cucumber, green onions, parsley, jicama,

and jalapeno. Toss gently with the squid and the olive oil dressing mixture. Chill until serving.

Nutrition

236 calories; protein 10.5g; carbohydrates 10.9g; fat 14.6g; cholesterol 132.2mg; sodium 51.6mg

Lemon Rice with Vegetables

Prep:20 mins
Cook:25 mins
Servings:4

Ingredients

2 tablespoons butter
1 tablespoon olive oil
4 green onions, chopped, white and green parts separated
1 teaspoon lemon zest
1 cup long grain rice
salt and ground black pepper to taste
1 cup low-sodium vegetable broth
1 cup 2% milk
3 tablespoons lemon juice
3 cloves garlic, minced
1 tablespoon chopped fresh dill
¼ teaspoon turmeric powder

Directions

Melt butter and oil together in a nonstick pan over medium heat. Add white parts of green onions and cook for 1 minute. Stir in garlic and lemon zest. Cook and stir until fragrant, about 30 seconds. Add rice. Season with turmeric, salt, and pepper. Cook and stir for 1 minute.

2
Stir vegetable broth, milk, and lemon juice into the pan with the rice mixture and bring to a boil, about 5 minutes. Reduce heat to a simmer, cover the pan, and cook until liquid has evaporated, 18 to 20 minutes.

3

Remove pan from heat. Fluff rice using a fork and adjust seasonings accordingly. Garnish with green parts of green onions and chopped dill.

Nutrition

295 calories; protein 5.9g; carbohydrates 43.4g; fat 10.7g; cholesterol 20.1mg; sodium 160.8mg.

Hawaiian Rice

Prep:15 mins
Cook:30 mins
Additional:15 mins
Servings:4

Ingredients

warm water, as needed
3 chicken breasts, or more to taste
water, to cover
1 quart chicken broth
1 small onion, sliced thin
1 (16 ounce) package bean thread vermicelli noodles
3 cloves garlic, chopped
 slices fresh ginger, chopped
1 tablespoon patis (Philippine-style fish sauce)
3 bay leaves
salt and ground black pepper to taste
2 cups chopped bok choy
 tablespoon soy sauce

Directions

Put bean thread noodles in a large bowl. Pour enough warm water over the noodles to cover by an inch. Soak noodles until softened, about 15 minutes; drain. Cut noodles into shorter lengths as desired.
    2
Put chicken breasts in a large pot with enough water to cover by a few inches; bring to a boil and cook chicken until until no longer pink in the center and the juices run clear, 8 to 10 minutes. An instant-read thermometer inserted into the center should read at least 165 degrees F .

3

Remove chicken breasts to a cutting board and shred into strands with 2 forks; return shredded chicken to the pot of boiling water.

4

Pour chicken broth into the pot and reduce heat to medium-high; add onion, garlic, ginger, fish sauce, soy sauce, and bay leaves; season with salt and pepper. Bring liquid again to a boil and add the bean thread noodles; cook at a boil until the noodles are translucent, about 6 minutes.

5

Stir bok choy into the liquid; cook just until the leaves wilt slightly, 1 to 2 minutes.

Nutrition

563 calories; protein 70.6g; carbohydrates 29.4g; fat 20.8g; cholesterol 50.6mg; sodium 1532.9mg.

BAKED HADDOCK

Prep:10 mins
Cook:15 mins
Servings:4

Ingredients

¾ cup milk
2 teaspoons salt
¼ cup grated Parmesan cheese
4 haddock fillets
¼ cup butter, melted
¼ teaspoon ground dried thyme
¾ cup bread crumbs

Directions

Preheat oven to 500 degrees F .
  2
In a small bowl, combine the milk and salt. In a separate bowl, mix together the bread crumbs, Parmesan cheese, and thyme. Dip the haddock fillets in the milk, then press into the crumb mixture to coat. Place haddock fillets in a glass baking dish, and drizzle with melted butter.
  3
Bake on the top rack of the preheated oven until the fish flakes easily, about 15 minutes.

Nutrition

325 calories; protein 27.7g; carbohydrates 17g; fat 15.7g; cholesterol 103.3mg; sodium 1565.2mg.

Mexico Rice

Prep:20 mins
Cook:30 mins
Servings:8

Ingredients

3 tablespoons vegetable oil
1 ½ cups uncooked white rice
1 cup chopped green bell pepper
⅔ cup diced onion
1 teaspoon ground cumin
1 teaspoon chili powder
2 teaspoons salt
⅛ teaspoon powdered saffron
1 ½ (8 ounce) cans tomato sauce
3 cups water
1 clove garlic, minced

Directions

In a large saucepan, heat vegetable oil over a medium-low heat. Place the onions in the pan, and saute until golden.
   2
Add rice to pan, and stir to coat grains with oil. Mix in green bell pepper, cumin, chili powder, tomato sauce, salt, garlic, saffron, and water. Cover, bring to a boil, and then reduce heat to simmer. Cook for 30 to 40 minutes, or until rice is tender. Stir occasionally.

Nutrition

199 calories; protein 3.4g; carbohydrates 33.8g; fat 5.6g; sodium 809.4mg.

BEET SALAD

Prep:20 mins
Cook:45 mins
Servings:16

Ingredients

4 bunches fresh small beets, stems removed
2 tablespoons olive oil
2 tablespoons white wine vinegar
1 tablespoon honey
1 teaspoon dried thyme, crushed
½ cup vegetable oil
1 tablespoon lemon juice
salt and pepper to taste
2 medium heads Belgian endive
1 pound spring lettuce mix
1 cup crumbled feta cheese
2 tablespoons Dijon mustard

Directions

Preheat oven to 450 degrees F . Coat beets lightly with oil and roast
for approximately 45 minutes, or until tender. Allow to cool
thoroughly, then peel and dice.
    2
For the dressing, place lemon, vinegar, honey, mustard, and thyme in a
blender. While blender is running, gradually add 1/2 cup of oil. Season
to taste with salt and pepper. Place spring lettuce mix in a salad bowl,
pour desired amount of dressing over greens, and toss to coat.
    3

Rinse endive, tear off whole leaves, and pat dry. Arrange 3 leaves on each plate. Divide dressed salad greens among them, and top with diced beets and feta cheese.

Nutrition

166 calories; protein 4.2g; carbohydrates 14.9g; fat 10.8g; cholesterol 8.3mg; sodium 253.6mg.

Garlic Italian Bread

Prep:10 mins
Cook:15 mins
Servings:8

Ingredients

½ cup butter
1 ½ tablespoons garlic powder
1 (1 pound) loaf Italian bread, cut into 1/2 inch slices
1 tablespoon dried parsley
1 (8 ounce) package shredded mozzarella cheese

Directions

Preheat oven to 350 degrees F (175 degrees C).

2

In a small saucepan over medium heat, melt butter and mix with garlic powder and dried parsley.

3

Place Italian bread on a medium baking sheet. Using a basting brush, brush generously with the butter mixture.

4

Bake in the preheated oven approximately 10 minutes, until lightly toasted. Remove from heat. Sprinkle with mozzarella cheese and any remaining butter mixture. Return to oven approximately 5 minutes, or until cheese is melted and bread is lightly browned.

Nutrition

332 calories; protein 12.2g; carbohydrates 30.4g; fat 18g; cholesterol 48.4mg; sodium 587.6mg.

Berries Salad With Salmon

Servings: 4

Ingredients

8 cups washed and chopped green leaf lettuce
1 cup fresh blackberries
1 cup fresh raspberries
1 cup sliced fresh strawberries
⅓ cup honey mustard dressing
12 ounces cooked and chilled salmon, flaked into bite-sized chunks

Directions

Combine lettuce, salmon, blackberries, raspberries, and strawberries in a large bowl and toss gently to combine.
   2
Drizzle salad with dressing and toss gently to coat.

Nutrition

268 calories; protein 19.5g; carbohydrates 18.7g; fat 13.7g; cholesterol 43.1mg; sodium 180.7mg

Garlic Steak Kebobs

Prep Time15 minutes
Cook Time15 minutes

INGREDIENTS

1 cup mushrooms
1 green bell pepper seeded, cored and diced into 1 inch pieces
1 red onion cut into 1 inch pieces
salt and pepper to taste
3 tablespoons butter
1 teaspoon minced garlic
2 teaspoons olive oil
1 tablespoon chopped parsley
1 pound beef sirloin cut into 1 inch pieces

DIRECTIONS

Heat a grill or indoor grill pan to medium high heat.
Thread the beef, mushrooms, pepper and onion onto skewers.
Brush the meat and vegetables with olive oil and season generously
with salt and pepper.
Place the kabobs onto the grill and cook for 4-5 minutes per side.
Melt the butter in a small pan over medium low. Add the garlic and
cook for 1 minute.
Remove the pan from the heat and stir in the parsley and salt and
pepper to taste.
Brush the garlic butter all over the steak kabobs, then serve.
Broiler Directions: Prepare the skewers as directed and place on a
sheet pan coated with cooking spray. Broil for 5 minutes per side.
Continue with the recipe as directed.

NUTRITION

Calories: 253kcal | Carbohydrates: 4g | Protein: 25g | Fat: 14g | Satur
ated

Fat: 7g | Cholesterol: 84mg | Sodium: 143mg | Potassium: 550mg | F
iber: 1g | Sugar: 2g | Vitamin A: 370IU | Vitamin

C: 26.5mg | Calcium: 34mg | Iron: 2.3mg

Avocado - Shrimp Salad

Prep:25 mins
Servings:4

Ingredients

2 avocados - peeled, pitted, and cubed
2 tomatoes, diced
1 pound cooked salad shrimp
1 pinch salt and pepper to taste
2 tablespoons lime juice
1 small sweet onion, chopped

Directions

Stir together avocadoes, tomatoes, onion, and shrimp in a large bowl.
Season to taste with salt and pepper. Stir in lime juice. Serve cold.

Nutrition

319 calories; protein 29.1g; carbohydrates 14.9g; fat 17.1g; cholesterol
196.4mg; sodium 203.4mg.

Tzatziki

Prep:20 mins
Additional:6 hrs
Servings:32

Ingredients

32 ounces plain yogurt
¼ cup extra virgin olive oil
5 cloves garlic, minced
3 tablespoons distilled white vinegar
1 large English cucumber, peeled and shredded
salt to taste

Directions

Place a cheese cloth over a medium bowl and strain the yogurt 6 hours
in the refrigerator, or over night.
  2
Drain as much excess liquid from the cucumber and garlic as possible.
  3
In a large bowl, mix together the yogurt, cucumber, garlic, vinegar,
olive oil and salt. Stir until a thick mixture has formed.

Nutrition

35 calories; protein 1.6g; carbohydrates 2.4g; fat 2.2g; cholesterol
1.7mg; sodium 19.9mg.

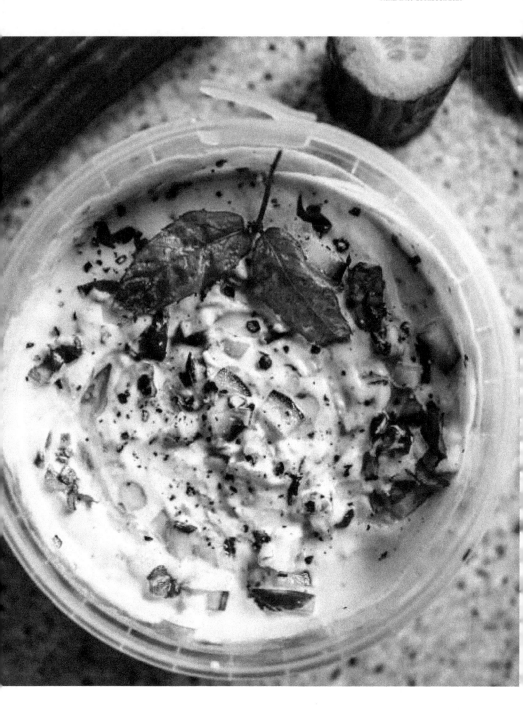

Daikon Salad

Servings: 16

Ingredients

large daikon (about 1 lb.), peeled, thinly sliced into 3"-long matchsticks
¾tsp. kosher salt, divided
1red finger or Fresno chile, seeds removed, finely chopped
2garlic cloves, finely chopped
2Tbsp. toasted sesame oil
2Tbsp. unseasoned rice vinegar
1Tbsp. granulated sugar
½–1tsp. store-bought or homemade chile crisp (optional)
Toasted white and/or black sesame seeds (for serving)

Directions

1

Toss daikon and ½ tsp. salt in a medium bowl; let sit 30 minutes. Transfer to a dish towel and squeeze out excess moisture.

2

Meanwhile, whisk chile, garlic, oil, vinegar, sugar, and remaining ¼ tsp. salt in a large bowl and let sit 25-30 minutes.

3

Add daikon to bowl and massage dressing into daikon. Let sit at least 30 minutes and up to 6 hours (cover and chill if holding longer than 1 hour).

4

To serve, stir in desired amount of chile crisp if using and top with sesame seeds.

Orzo Salad

Prep:1 hr 10 mins
Cook:10 mins
Servings:6

Ingredients

1 ½ cups uncooked orzo pasta
½ teaspoon lemon pepper
1 tomato, seeded and chopped
1 cucumber, seeded and chopped
1 red onion, chopped
 (2 ounce) can black olives, drained
2 (6 ounce) cans marinated artichoke hearts
¼ cup chopped fresh parsley
1 tablespoon lemon juice
½ teaspoon dried oregano
1 cup crumbled feta cheese

Directions

Bring a large pot of lightly salted water to a boil. Add pasta and cook
for 8 to 10 minutes or until al dente; drain. Drain artichoke hearts,
reserving liquid.
    2
In large bowl combine pasta, artichoke hearts, tomato, cucumber,
onion, feta, olives, parsley, lemon juice, oregano and lemon pepper.
Toss and chill for 60 minutes in refrigerator.
    3
Just before serving, drizzle reserved artichoke marinade over salad.

Nutrition

:

326 calories; protein 13.1g; carbohydrates 48.7g; fat 10.2g; cholesterol 22.3mg; sodium 615.2mg.

Colourful Papaya Salad

Prep:15 mins
Total:15 mins
Servings:6

Ingredients

1 large mango - peeled, seeded and halved
1 avocado - peeled, pitted and diced
3 tablespoons balsamic vinegar
¼ cup blanched slivered almonds
1 teaspoon brown sugar
1 medium papaya - peeled, seeded and halved
1 head romaine lettuce, torn into bite-size pieces
1 tablespoon butter
salt to taste

Directions

Place half of the mango and half of the papaya into the container of a food processor or blender along with balsamic vinegar. Puree until smooth, and set aside.

2

Melt butter in a small skillet over medium heat. Add almonds, and cook stirring constantly until lightly browned. Add brown sugar, and stir to coat. Remove from heat, and pour candied almonds onto a piece of waxed paper, separating any clumps. Set aside to cool.

3

Just before serving, place romaine lettuce in a large serving bowl. Cube remaining mango and papaya halves, and toss gently with avocado and lettuce. Drizzle the pureed fruit over the salad and lightly salt. Sprinkle with candied almonds, and serve immediately.

Nutrition

148 calories; protein 2.7g; carbohydrates 16g; fat 9.4g; cholesterol 5.1mg; sodium 24.6mg.

MEDITERRANEAN TUNA STICKS

Prep:10 mins
Cook:11 mins
Additional:30 mins
Servings:4

Ingredients

¼ cup orange juice
1 tablespoon lemon juice
2 tablespoons chopped fresh parsley
1 clove garlic, minced
½ teaspoon chopped fresh oregano
2 tablespoons olive oil
½ teaspoon ground black pepper
4 (4 ounce) tuna steaks
¼ cup soy sauce

Directions

In a large non-reactive dish, mix together the orange juice, soy sauce, olive oil, lemon juice, parsley, garlic, oregano, and pepper. Place the tuna steaks in the marinade and turn to coat. Cover, and refrigerate for at least 30 minutes.

2

Preheat grill for high heat.

3

Lightly oil grill grate. Cook the tuna steaks for 5 to 6 minutes, then turn and baste with the marinade. Cook for an additional 5 minutes, or to desired doneness. Discard any remaining marinade.

Nutrition

200 calories; protein 27.4g; carbohydrates 3.7g; fat 7.9g; cholesterol 50.6mg; sodium 944.6mg.

Corn Salad

Prep:15 mins
Cook:10 mins
Additional:45 mins
Servings:6

Ingredients

6 ears freshly shucked corn
½ bunch fresh cilantro, chopped, or more to taste
1 green pepper, diced
¼ cup diced red onion
 teaspoons olive oil, or to taste
2 Roma (plum) tomatoes, diced
salt and ground black pepper to taste

Directions

Preheat an outdoor grill for medium heat; lightly oil the grate.
    2
Cook the corn on the preheated grill, turning occasionally, until the
corn is tender and specks of black appear, about 10 minutes; set aside
until just cool enough to handle. Slice the kernels off of the cob and
place into a bowl.
    3
Combine the warm corn kernels with the green pepper, diced tomato,
onion, cilantro, and olive oil. Season with salt and pepper; toss until
evenly mixed. Set aside for at least 30 minutes to allow flavors to blend
before serving.

Nutrition

:

103 calories; protein 3.4g; carbohydrates 19.7g; fat 2.8g; sodium 43.4mg.

EGG WHITE AND AVOCADO SALAD

Prep:15 mins
Total:15 mins
Servings:4

Ingredients

2 cups fresh baby spinach
1 pinch ground black pepper to taste
6 hard-boiled egg whites, chopped into 1/2-inch pieces
2 tablespoons light mayonnaise
2 tablespoons sliced black olives
1 avocado - peeled, pitted, and cut into 1/2-inch pieces
2 teaspoons freshly squeezed lemon juice
½ teaspoon sea salt

Directions

Place spinach, avocado, egg whites, and mayonnaise in a large bowl;
gently toss to coat. Add celery, olives, lemon juice, salt, and pepper;
lightly toss to combine.

Nutrition

141 calories; protein 6.9g; carbohydrates 6.9g; fat 10.4g; cholesterol
2.6mg; sodium 412.8mg.

Avocado and Mango Salad

Prep:30 mins
Servings:8

Ingredients

Dressing:
½ cup white wine vinegar
¼ cup sunflower seed oil
ground black pepper
4 ripe avocados, cubed
1 teaspoon white sugar
2 mango, cubed
lemons, juiced
2 teaspoons dry mustard
1 head iceberg lettuce, torn, or to taste
1 ½ cups walnut halves
6 slices crispy cooked bacon, crumbled

Directions

Combine vinegar, oil, sugar, mustard, and pepper in a bowl.
Refrigerate dressing until ready to serve.
  2
Place avocados, mangoes, and lemon juice in a bowl. Mix gently until
just combined.
  3
Place lettuce in a large bowl or platter. Add avocado-mango mixture,
walnuts, bacon, and the dressing. Toss and serve.

Nutrition

486 calories; protein 10.1g; carbohydrates 28.6g; fat 40.6g; cholesterol 9.9mg; sodium 225.4mg.

Fish Salad

Prep:15 mins
Total:15 mins
Servings:4

Ingredients

1 (5 ounce) can tuna, drained
1 tablespoon chopped fresh parsley
⅛ teaspoon ground black pepper
½ cup mayonnaise
½ teaspoon lemon juice
¼ cup chopped onion
¼ cup chopped celery
¼ teaspoon garlic powder
⅛ teaspoon salt
paprika to taste

Directions

In a large bowl, combine the tuna, celery, onion, mayonnaise, lemon juice, parsley, garlic powder, salt and pepper. Mix well and refrigerate until chilled. Sprinkle with paprika if desired.

Nutrition

240 calories; protein 8.5g; carbohydrates 2.3g; fat 22.1g; cholesterol 19.9mg; sodium 251.6mg.

HEALTHY BBQ SALAD

Prep:15 mins
Cook:12 mins
Additional:8 mins
Servings:8

Ingredients

2 skinless, boneless chicken breast halves
1 head red leaf lettuce, rinsed and torn
1 fresh tomato, chopped
1 bunch cilantro, chopped
½ cup barbeque sauce
1 (15.25 ounce) can whole kernel corn, drained
1 (15 ounce) can black beans, drained
1 (2.8 ounce) can French fried onions
1 head green leaf lettuce, rinsed and torn
½ cup Ranch dressing

Directions

Preheat the grill for high heat.
    2
Lightly oil the grill grate. Place chicken on the grill, and cook 6
minutes per side, or until juices run clear. Remove from heat, cool, and
slice.
    3
In a large bowl, mix the red leaf lettuce, green leaf lettuce, tomato,
cilantro, corn, and black beans. Top with the grilled chicken slices and
French fried onions.
    4
In a small bowl, mix the Ranch dressing and barbeque sauce. Serve on
the side as a dipping sauce, or toss with the salad to coat.

Nutrition

301 calories; protein 12.2g; carbohydrates 32.3g; fat 14.4g; cholesterol 20.8mg; sodium 805.4mg.

SALMON PATE'

Prep:30 mins
Additional:30 mins
Servings:8

Ingredients

1 (7 ounce) can salmon, drained, flaked and bones removed
1 (8 ounce) package cream cheese, softened
1 tablespoon lemon juice
2 teaspoons grated onion
1 teaspoon prepared horseradish
1 tablespoon chopped fresh parsley

Directions

In a medium bowl, mix together the salmon, cream cheese, horseradish, lemon juice, and onion. Chill if necessary until firm enough to handle, then form into a ball. Roll in parsley and/or pecans. Refrigerate until serving. Serve with assorted crackers.

Nutrition

191 calories; protein 8.6g; carbohydrates 2.1g; fat 16.9g; cholesterol 41.6mg; sodium 173.4mg.

Aragula Salad

Prep Time 5 minutes
Total Time 5 minutes
Servings 2 servings
Calories 203 kcal

Ingredients

2 tablespoons fresh lemon juice
1/2 teaspoon freshly ground black pepper
1/2 teaspoon kosher salt
1 teaspoon honey
4 cups arugula
1/4 cup shaved Parmesan cheese
2 tablespoons olive oil

DIRECTIONS

In a large bowl, whisk together the olive oil, lemon juice, honey, and salt and pepper.
Add the arugula to the bowl and toss. Top with the shaved Parmesan and more pepper taste. Makes 4 cups.

Shish Tawook

Prep:30 mins
Cook:10 mins
Additional:4 hrs
Servings:6

Ingredients

¼ cup lemon juice
¾ cup plain yogurt
4 cloves garlic, minced
2 teaspoons tomato paste
1 ½ teaspoons salt
1 teaspoon dried oregano
¼ cup vegetable oil
¼ teaspoon ground allspice
¼ teaspoon ground black pepper
⅛ teaspoon ground cardamom
2 pounds skinless, boneless chicken breast halves - cut into 2 inch pieces
¼ teaspoon ground cinnamon
2 onions, cut into large chunks
1 cup chopped fresh flat-leaf parsley
1 large green bell pepper, cut into large chunks

Directions

Whisk together the lemon juice, vegetable oil, plain yogurt, garlic, tomato paste, salt, oregano, pepper, allspice, cinnamon, and cardamom in a large bowl; add the chicken and toss to coat. Transfer the chicken mixture into a large plastic bag; refrigerate at least 4 hours.

2

Preheat an outdoor grill for medium-high heat and lightly oil grate. Thread the chicken, onions, and pepper onto metal skewers. Cook on preheated grill until the chicken is golden and no longer pink in the center, about 5 minutes each side. Sprinkle the parsley over the skewers.

Nutrition

299 calories; protein 34.3g; carbohydrates 9.8g; fat 13.4g; cholesterol 88mg; sodium 701.5mg.

Sensational Moose Jerky

Prep:1 hr
Cook:12 hrs
Servings:6

Ingredients

3 cups soy sauce
3 pounds rump roast
4 fluid ounces hickory-flavored liquid smoke
3 cups packed brown sugar

Directions

Slice roast into slabs approximately 1/4 inch thick, (Note: you can have this done at the grocery store or butcher). Trim off all of the fat from the edges. Cut the slabs into pencil-like strips (about 1/4 inch wide), and about 4 inches long.

2

In a large bowl, combine the soy sauce, brown sugar and hickory-flavored liquid smoke; blend well. Place all of the meat into the bowl of marinade. Cover and place in refrigerator for at least 30 minutes.

3

Place the meat in a food dehydrator for about 12 to 20 hours, depending how dry you like your jerky. Rotate the trays after 6 hours. For example: Bottom tray on top, top tray on bottom, second tray from bottom to be second tray from top, and so on.

Nutrition

1129 calories; protein 52.9g; carbohydrates 117.6g; fat 50.5g; cholesterol 138.3mg; sodium 7357.3mg.

Turmeric and Broccoli Soup

Prep:25 mins
Cook:30 mins
Additional:10 mins
Servings:6

Ingredients

1 ½ pounds broccoli florets and stems
3 tablespoons extra-virgin olive oil
1 carrot, diced
1 large clove garlic, minced
1 onion, diced
1 ½ tablespoons minced fresh ginger
1 teaspoon turmeric powder
½ cup diced red bell pepper
½ teaspoon cracked black pepper
¾ cup plain yogurt
1 (32 ounce) carton low-sodium chicken broth

Directions

Remove broccoli florets from stems and set aside. Trim leaves and set aside. Cut away and discard the tough outer portion of the stems. Dice the remaining cores.
    2
Turn on a multi-functional pressure cooker,

Nutrition

151 calories; protein 7.4g; carbohydrates 14.5g; fat 8g; cholesterol 4.4mg; sodium 138.7mg.

Falafel

Prep:20 mins
Cook:10 mins
Additional:12 hrs
Servings:6

Ingredients

1 cup dry garbanzo beans
½ yellow onion, diced
4 cloves minced garlic
1 tablespoon all-purpose flour
½ cup chopped fresh flat-leaf parsley
2 teaspoons lemon juice
1 ½ teaspoons salt
oil for frying
½ teaspoon ground coriander
¼ teaspoon baking soda
⅛ teaspoon cayenne pepper
1 teaspoon ground cumin

Directions

Wrap onion in cheese cloth and squeeze out as much moisture as possible. Set aside. Place garbanzo beans, parsley, garlic, cumin, coriander, salt, and baking soda in a food processor. Process until the mixture is coarsely pureed. Mix garbanzo bean mixture and onion together in a bowl. Stir in the flour and egg. Shape mixture into four large patties and let stand for 15 minutes.
Preheat an oven to 400 degrees F (200 degrees C).

Heat olive oil in a large, oven-safe skillet over medium-high heat. Place the patties in the skillet; cook until golden brown, about 3 minutes on each side.

Transfer skillet to the preheated oven and bake until heated through, about 10 minutes.

Nutrition

271 calories; protein 7.1g; carbohydrates 24.4g; fat 16.9g; sodium 646.4mg

Mint Pesto Zucchini Noodles

Prep Time25 minutes
Total Time25 minutes
Servings4

Ingredients

1/4 cup sliced almonds, toasted
1 cup mint leaves
1/4 cup extra-virgin olive oil
1/4 cup fresh dill
1 clove garlic chopped
1/4 cup grated Parmesan cheese
2 tbsp lemon juice
3 medium zucchini
Salt and pepper to taste

Directions

For the almonds:
Heat oven to 350°F. Place slivered almonds in a single layer on a baking sheet, and toast for 8 minutes, or until they have browned slightly and just become fragrant. Remove the sheet from the oven and immediately place almonds on a plate or in a bowl.
For the mint pesto:
Add mint leaves, dill, and garlic to the bowl of a food processor and process until the herbs are finely broken up. Add olive oil, Parmesan, lemon juice, and salt and pepper and process until creamy.
For the zucchini noodles:
Slice the very ends off of three zucchini and spiralize using the fine spiralizer blade (or your blade of choice). Add the zucchini noodles to a large mixing bowl and pour in the pesto sauce. Toss to combine.

Top with additional Parmesan, dill, mint, and/or toasted almonds for serving, along with your favorite protein if making this a full meal.

Nutrition

Calories: 169kcal | Carbohydrates: 6.5g | Protein: 4.5g | Fat: 15.4g | S aturated
Fat: 2.9g | Cholesterol: 4mg | Sodium: 150mg | Potassium: 452mg | Fiber: 2.2g | Sugar: 2.8g | Calcium: 70mg | Iron: 1.1mg

Grilled Teriyaki Tuna

Prep:5 mins
Cook:10 mins
Additional:30 mins
Servings:4

Ingredients

1 cup teriyaki sauce
¾ cup olive oil
1 teaspoon ground black pepper
2 tablespoons minced garlic
4 (4 ounce) fillets yellowfin tuna

Directions

In a large resealable plastic bag, combine the teriyaki sauce, oil, garlic,
and pepper. Place the tuna fillets in the bag. Seal the bag with as little
air in it as possible. Give the mix a good shake, to ensure the tuna
fillets are well coated. Marinate for 30 minutes in the refrigerator.
Meanwhile, preheat an outdoor grill for high heat, and lightly oil grate.
Remove tuna from marinade, and place on grill. For rare tuna, grill for
5 minutes on each side. For medium, grill 6 to 8 minutes per side. For
well done, grill for 8 to 10 minutes per side.

Nutrition

551 calories; protein 30.7g; carbohydrates 12.9g; fat 41.6g; cholesterol
50.6mg; sodium 2802.5mg.

Chicken Soup

Servings:2

Ingredients

2 cups water
1 zucchini, diced
1 boneless chicken breast half, cooked and diced
1 clove garlic, minced
½ teaspoon chicken broth base
2 carrots, chopped

Directions

Put cooked chicken meat and water in a large pot and bring to a boil.
Add the carrots, zucchini and garlic and simmer all together for 5 to 10 minutes.
Add the chicken broth and simmer for an additional 5 minutes. Serve.

Nutrition

150 calories; protein 17.1g; carbohydrates 10.8g; fat 4.6g; cholesterol 41.4mg; sodium 288.5mg.

Tandoori salmon kebabs

Serves: 2 (Not suitable for home freezing)
Prep time: 15 minutes plus marinating time
Cooking time: 10 minutes

INGREDIENTS

2 x 115g (4oz) salmon steaks, skinned
3 small new potatoes
½ teaspoon ground turmeric
1 tbsp chopped fresh mint or coriander
Small piece fresh ginger, peeled and grated
Finely grated zest and juice of ½ lime or lemon
½ teaspoon garam masala
1 clove garlic, crushed
4 tbsp fat-free Greek yoghurt

Directions

Cut the salmon into large, bite-sized chunks. Steam or boil the
potatoes until just tender then drain, cool and halve.
In a medium bowl, mix together the ginger, lemon, spices, garlic, mint
and yoghurt. Stir in the fish and potatoes, cover and marinate in the
fridge for at least one hour.
Thread the fish cubes and the potatoes onto wooden skewers and grill
or barbecue for 5 minutes, turning until evenly browned.
Serve immediately with brown basmati rice, rocket or watercress, and
lemon wedges.

Garlic Chicken Balls

Prep: 10 mins
Cook: 10 mins
Servings: 3

Ingredients

500g chicken mince
2 eggs
4 tablespoons butter
2 cups breadcrumbs
3 tablespoons garlic
Cooking oil
1.5 tablespoons parsley

Directions

Melt butter in a small microwave-safe bowl. Mix in crushed garlic and chopped parsley and stir well. Allow your garlic butter mixture to set in refrigerator or freezer until it is firm. It takes 30-60 minutes in the freezer, so you may want to make the day before.
Roll chicken mince into balls, around 2 inches in diameter.
When the garlic butter is set, cut into cubes. Insert one cube of garlic butter into the centre of each mince ball and smooth over with mince, to ensure the butter cube is completely encased.
Whisk eggs in a bowl. Dip chicken balls in egg mixture, then coat generously in breadcrumbs. Repeat with all the chicken balls.

Winter Citrus Salad

Prep:30 mins

Servings:6

Ingredients

Dressing:

½ cup canola oil

¼ cup apple cider vinegar

½ cup white sugar

2 tablespoons sesame oil

2 tablespoons toasted sesame seeds

1 teaspoon minced garlic

2 tablespoons poppy seeds

½ teaspoon ground paprika

2 tablespoons minced onion

Salad:

1 (12 ounce) bag mixed salad greens

¼ cup chopped green onions

1 (8 ounce) can mandarin oranges, drained

½ cup toasted sliced almonds

¼ cup crumbled Gorgonzola cheese

½ cup grape tomatoes

Directions

Combine canola oil, sugar, apple cider vinegar, sesame oil, onion, poppy seeds, sesame seeds, garlic, and paprika in a jar. Close and shake jar until dressing is well mixed.

Place salad greens in a large bowl. Pour in half of the dressing; toss to mix. Arrange mandarin oranges, grape tomatoes, almonds, Gorgonzola cheese, and green onions on top.

Nutrition

404 calories; protein 5.2g; carbohydrates 26.3g; fat 31.7g; cholesterol 6mg; sodium 75.7mg.

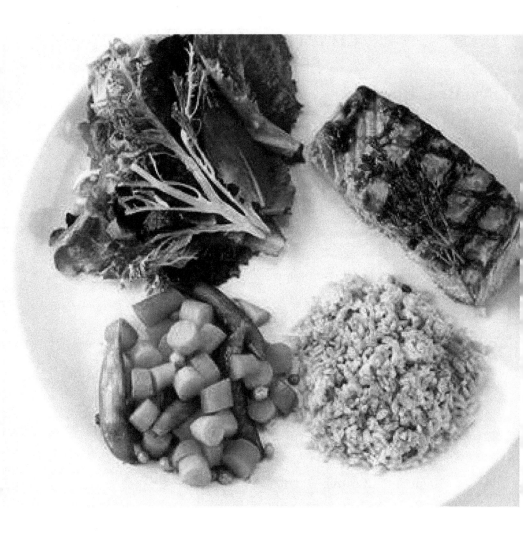

CHAPTER 3: DINNER

Beef Burritos

Prep:30 mins
Cook:20 mins
Servings:6

Ingredients

6 ounces sliced jalapeno peppers
1 tomato, diced
1 green bell pepper, diced
1 red bell pepper, diced
1 onion, diced
1 ½ tablespoons hot sauce
¼ teaspoon ground cayenne pepper
1 (4 ounce) can chopped green chile peppers
1 pound ground beef
1 (14 ounce) can refried beans
6 (10 inch) flour tortillas
1 (10 ounce) bag shredded lettuce
1 (1 ounce) package burrito seasoning
1 (8 ounce) package shredded sharp Cheddar cheese
1 (8 ounce) container sour cream

Directions

Mix jalapeno peppers, tomato, green chile peppers, green bell pepper, red bell pepper, onion, hot sauce, and cayenne pepper together in a large bowl.

Cook beef in a large skillet over medium-high heat, stirring to break up clumps, about 5 minutes. Drain excess grease. Add jalapeno pepper mixture and burrito seasoning; cook, covered, stirring occasionally, until flavors combine, about 10 minutes.

Pour refried beans into a saucepan over medium-low heat. Cook and stir until heated through, about 5 minutes.

Warm each tortilla in the microwave until soft, 15 to 20 seconds. Spread a layer of refried beans on top. Divide beef mixture among tortillas. Top with lettuce, sour cream, and Cheddar cheese. Fold in opposing edges of each tortilla and roll up into a burrito.

Nutrition

723 calories; protein 34g; carbohydrates 59.9g; fat 38.9g; cholesterol 107.5mg; sodium 2042.5mg.

Pork Medallions

Prep: 30 mins
Total:30 mins
Servings:4

Ingredients

1 cup Holland House® Sake Cooking Wine
2 tablespoons brown sugar, not packed
1 teaspoon cornstarch
1 ½ pounds pork tenderloin
2 tablespoons butter
1 teaspoon toasted sesame oil
Minced green onion (garnish)
2 tablespoons toasted sesame seeds

Directions

Combine sake cooking wine, sugar, sesame oil and cornstarch. Stir to
dissolve cornstarch; set aside.
Cut pork into 1/2-inch slices; season with salt and pepper to taste.
Press half the sesame seeds onto one side of each medallion. Melt
butter in 12-inch saute pan. Cook pork, seed side down, over medium-
high heat until lightly browned, about 8 minutes. While cooking, press
remaining sesame seeds onto tops of medallions. Turn over and
continue to cook 5 minutes. Increase heat to high, add sauce and cook
3 minutes or until sauce bubbles and thickens slightly. Serve pork
medallions drizzled with sake sauce. Sprinkle with any remaining
sesame seeds and green onion.

Nutrition

290 calories, 34g protein, 8g carb, 13g fat (5g sat. fat), 110mg chol, 320mg sodium, 0g fiber

Iberian Shrimp Fritters

Ingredients:

100 grams of fresh shrimp.
1 cup water, approximately 250 ml
100 grams of wheat flour.
100 grams of chickpea flour.
1 spring onion.
Parsley.
Olive oil for frying shrimp omelettes
A little bit of salt.

Directions

The recipe for shrimp omelettes is very simple. Start making the dough in a bowl, we will overturn wheat flour and chickpea flour first, then we will include minced scallions into thin pieces and very small with parsley, and finally add a pinch of salt, shrimp and water. After mixing all, already we have the dough! You must stay a fairly liquid mass.

Once we have the mass of shrimp omelettes, the next is frying. To do this we fill a large pan with enough oil, about one finger, and when hot, with a ladle, add the mixture gently spreading it, and we make cuts with a knife to make them finer and fry before. When the shrimp tortilla is golden brown on one side, we turn to the other side too browned and removed on a plate with kitchen paper to absorb the oil. Serve accompanied by a glass of Manzanilla.

Mushrooms Tacos

Prep:30 mins
Cook:10 mins
Servings:8

Ingredients

4 tablespoons olive oil
1 ½ cups chopped onion
1 pound ground venison
1 (8 ounce) package mushrooms, finely chopped or pulsed in a food processor
1 package taco seasoning
3 cloves garlic, minced
1 cup shredded cabbage
2 tablespoons chopped cilantro
salt and ground black pepper to taste
8 corn tortillas
2 tablespoons lime juice
1 (8 ounce) jar salsa, or as desired
¼ cup crumbled blue cheese, or to taste

Directions

Heat olive oil in a saute pan over medium-high heat. Add onions and cook about 3 minutes. Add garlic and cook 2 minutes more. Add venison and mushrooms; saute until venison is cooked through, 5 to 7 minutes more. Season with taco seasoning.
Toss cabbage, lime juice, cilantro, salt, and pepper together in a bowl. Place about 2 tablespoons cabbage mixture onto a tortilla and top with about 2 tablespoons meat mixture. Top with salsa and blue cheese. Repeat with remaining fillings, tortillas, and toppings.

Nutrition

238 calories; protein 15.8g; carbohydrates 21.5g; fat 10.1g; cholesterol 45.9mg; sodium 596.2mg.

Mussels with Saffron

Prep:35 mins
Cook:35 mins
Servings:6

Ingredients

2 pounds mussels, cleaned and debearded
1 ¼ cups white wine
3 tablespoons margarine
1 tablespoon olive oil
1 onion, chopped
1 ½ cups water
1 clove garlic, crushed
1 leek, bulb only, chopped
1 ½ tablespoons all-purpose flour
6 saffron threads
1 ¼ cups chicken broth
1 tablespoon chopped fresh parsley
½ teaspoon fenugreek seeds, finely crushed
salt and pepper to taste
2 tablespoons whipping cream

Directions

Place saffron threads in a small bowl, and cover with 1 tablespoon boiling water. Set aside.
Scrub mussels clean in several changes of fresh water and pull off beards. Discard any mussels that are cracked or do not close tightly when tapped. Put mussels into a saucepan with wine and water. Cover and cook over high heat, shaking pan frequently, 5-7 minutes or until shells open. Remove mussels, discarding any which remain closed. Strain liquid through a fine sieve and reserve.

Heat butter and oil in a saucepan. Add onion, garlic, leek and fenugreek and cook gently 5 minutes. Stir in flour and cook 1 minute. Add saffron mixture, 2-1/2 cups of reserved cooking liquid and chicken broth. Bring to a boil, cover and simmer gently for 15 minutes.

Meanwhile, keep 8 mussels in shells and remove remaining mussels from shells. Add all mussels to soup and stir in chopped parsley, salt, pepper and cream. Heat through 2-4 minutes. Garnish with parsley sprigs, if desired, and serve hot.

Nutrition

205 calories; protein 9.7g; carbohydrates 9g; fat 10.4g; cholesterol 27mg; sodium 343.1mg.

Lamb with Spinach

Prep:30 mins
Cook:30 mins
Servings:4

Ingredients

20 potatoes, halved
2 cloves garlic, minced
2 tablespoons brown sugar
1 cup red wine
4 (6 ounce) lamb shoulder steaks
salt and pepper to taste
1 tablespoon butter
1 tablespoon cumin seeds
2 bunches fresh spinach, cleaned
¼ cup sour cream
2 tablespoons softened butter
1 tablespoon vegetable oil

Directions

Place potatoes into a large saucepan and cover with salted water. Bring to a boil, then reduce heat to medium-low, cover, and simmer until tender, about 15 minutes. Drain and allow to steam dry for a minute or two.

Melt the butter in a saucepan over medium heat. Stir in the garlic, and cook for 3 to 4 minutes until the aroma of the garlic has mellowed. Add the brown sugar and red wine, then bring to a boil over medium-high heat. Allow to boil for 5 minutes, then remove from the heat, cover, and keep warm.

Meanwhile, season the lamb steaks with salt and pepper to taste. Press the cumin seeds into the steaks on both sides. Heat the vegetable oil in a large skillet over medium-high heat. Add the steaks, and cook on both sides until cooked to your desired degree of doneness, about 4 minutes per side for medium. Remove the steaks to rest in a warm spot. Place the spinach into the hot skillet, season to taste with salt and pepper, and cook until the spinach has wilted.

Mash the potatoes with the sour cream and butter; season to taste with salt and pepper. To serve, mound a serving of mashed potatoes onto the center of a dinner plate. Top with the spinach and a lamb steak. Strain the red wine sauce overtop.

Nutrition

1063 calories; protein 43.3g; carbohydrates 96.5g; fat 53g; cholesterol 151.6mg; sodium 341.7mg.

Mussels with Herbed Butter on Grill

Prep:10 mins
Cook:25 mins
Servings:4

Ingredients

1/4 cup (1/2 stick) unsalted butter
3 tablespoons chopped fresh parsley
3 pounds mussels, rinsed and scrubbed
Coarse salt and ground pepper
2 lemons

Directions

Heat a grill or grill pan to medium-high. Clean and lightly oil hot grill.
In a small pot, melt butter over medium. Remove from heat and stir in
parsley; set aside.
Working in batches if necessary, place mussels on grill in a single layer.
Place lemons, halved and lightly oiled, on grill, cut side down.
Grill until mussels open and lemons are warmed through and
browned, 5 minutes. With tongs, transfer mussels as they open to a
large platter. (Discard unopened mussels.) Pour herb butter over
mussels; sprinkle with salt and pepper. Serve with lemons.

White Fish Soup

PREP TIME10 mins
COOK TIME20 mins
SERVINGS4 servings

Ingredients

6 tablespoons extra virgin olive oil
1 medium onion, chopped (about 1 1/2 cups)
3 large garlic cloves, minced
1/8 teaspoon freshly ground black pepper
2/3 cup fresh parsley, chopped
1 1/2 cups of fresh chopped tomato (about 1 medium sized tomato)
OR 1 14-ounce can of whole or crushed tomatoes with their juices
1/2 cup dry white wine (like Sauvignon blanc)
1 1/2 pound fish fillets (use a firm white fish such as halibut, cod, red
snapper, or sea bass), cut into 2-inch pieces
Pinch of dry oregano
8 oz of clam juice
Pinch of dry thyme
1/8 teaspoon Tabasco sauce
1 teaspoon of salt

Directions

Sauté aromatics:
Heat olive oil in a large thick-bottomed pot over medium-high heat.
Add onion and sauté 4 minutes, add the garlic and cook a minute
more. Add parsley and stir 2 minutes. Add tomato and tomato paste,
and gently cook for 10 minutes or so.
Finish soup:
Add clam juice, dry white wine, and fish. Bring to a simmer and
simmer until the fish is cooked through and easily flakes apart, about 3

to 5 minutes. Add seasoning —salt, pepper, oregano, thyme, Tabasco. Add more salt and pepper to taste. Ladle into bowls and serve. Great served with crusty bread for dipping in the fish stew broth.

Fajita Beef

Cook:8 mins
Servings:4

Ingredients

1 (1 ounce) package fajita seasoning mix
1 pound boneless beef top round steak
1 medium red or yellow bell pepper, cut into strips
1 medium green bell pepper, cut into strips
1 medium onion, cut into 1/4-inch slices
eynolds Wrap® Heavy Duty Aluminum Foil
8 (8 inch) flour tortillas
1 tablespoon vegetable oil
Salsa

Directions

Prepare fajita seasoning mix following package directions and pour over steak. Cover with Reynolds Wrap® Heavy Duty Aluminum Foil and marinate steak 1 to 2 hours.

Make a grill pan by shaping two layers of foil over the outside of 13x9x2inch baking pan. Remove foil and crimp the edges to form a tight rim, making a pan with one inch sides. Place on cookie sheet. Preheat grill to high. Remove steak from marinade discard marinade. Add peppers, onion and oil to foil pan. Slide foil pan from cookie sheet onto grill and place steak beside pan on grill.

Grill 8 to 10 minutes on high in covered grill. Stir vegetables and turn steak after 5 minutes. Slide foil pan from grill onto cookie sheet. Slice grilled steak into thin strips.

Wrap tortillas in foil add to grill to heat while slicing steak. Serve beef, peppers and onions wrapped in warm tortillas with salsa.

Salmon Stuffed Pasta

Prep:15 mins
Cook:35 mins
Servings:8

Ingredients

2 (9 ounce) packages cheese tortellini
1 ¼ cups milk
1 bay leaf
2 whole cloves
1 pinch ground nutmeg
¼ cup butter
¼ small onion
1 red bell pepper, chopped
10 ounces fresh mushrooms, sliced
1 pound smoked salmon, chopped
½ pound fresh asparagus, trimmed and quartered
2 tablespoons all-purpose flour

Directions

Bring a large pot of water to a boil, and cook the tortellini for 8 minutes, or until al dente. Drain, and transfer to a large bowl.
In a saucepan over low heat, simmer the milk, onion, bay leaf, cloves, and nutmeg about 15 minutes. Remove from heat, and discard the onion, bay leaf, and cloves.
Melt 2 tablespoons butter in a large skillet over medium heat. Stir in the red bell pepper and asparagus, and cook about 3 minutes. Stir in the mushrooms, and continue cooking until tender. Mix in the smoked salmon, reduce heat to low, and cook until heated through.

Melt the remaining 2 tablespoons butter in a saucepan over medium heat, and slowly whisk in the flour until smooth. Thoroughly blend in the warmed milk. Stir into the skillet with the salmon mixture. Spoon the salmon and sauce mixture into the bowl with the cooked pasta, and toss to coat.

Nutrition

364 calories; protein 22.6g; carbohydrates 36.5g; fat 14.9g; cholesterol 59.4mg; sodium 745.9mg.

Hungarian Goulash

Prep:30 mins
Cook:4 hrs 15 mins
Servings:12

Ingredients

2 pounds cubed beef stew meat
2 onions, chopped
1 bunch celery, cut into 1/2 inch pieces
1 (15 ounce) can carrots, canned
2 quarts tomato juice
1 (15 ounce) can peas
2 bay leaves
1 (14.5 ounce) can green beans
2 teaspoons salt
2 (15 ounce) cans kidney beans
ground black pepper to taste

Directions

Place the beef stew meat and onions in a medium saucepan. Cook and stir over medium heat until evenly brown
In a large saucepan, place the meat, onions, tomato juice, celery, green beans, carrots, peas, bay leaves, salt and pepper. Bring to a boil.
Reduce heat and simmer 4 hours.
Stir in the kidney beans. Cook 15 minutes longer and serve warm.

Nutrition

353 calories; protein 20.9g; carbohydrates 32.8g; fat 15.4g; cholesterol 52.3mg; sodium 1345.9mg.

Broiled Shrimp

Prep:30 mins
Cook:15 mins
Servings:4

Ingredients

2 pounds medium shrimp, peeled and deveined
2 cloves garlic, minced
¼ cup dry white wine
3 green onions, chopped
½ cup butter, melted

Directions

Preheat broiler to 500 degrees .
Stir shrimp together with butter, garlic and wine. Place on a baking sheet and broil for 10 minutes. Sprinkle on scallions and broil for another 2 to 4 minutes, until shrimp are firm. Serve hot.

Nutrition

432 calories; protein 44.8g; carbohydrates 1.3g; fat 26.2g; cholesterol 419.7mg; sodium 672.4mg.

Turmeric Tilapia

Servings: 24

Ingredients

1 thumb
Ginger
1 Unit Lime
¼ ounce Cilantro
1 unit Shallot
2 clove Garlic
½ cup Jasmine Rice
1 tablespoon Brown Sugar
6 ounce Green Beans
11 ounce Tilapia
1 teaspoon Turmeric
¼ cup Shredded Coconut
1 unit Veggie Stock Concentrate

Directions

Wash and dry all produce (except green beans). Peel and grate or mince ginger. Zest and quarter lime (zest 1 lime; quarter both for 4 servings). Chop cilantro leaves and stems. Halve and peel shallot; mince one half (mince both halves for 4). Mince half the garlic (mince all the garlic for 4).

In a small pot, combine rice, ¾ cup water (1½ cups for 4 servings), brown sugar, and ½ tsp salt (1 tsp for 4). Bring to a boil, then cover and reduce to a low simmer. Cook until rice is tender, 16-18 minutes. Keep covered off heat until ready to serve.

Meanwhile, heat a large, preferably nonstick, pan over medium-high heat. Add coconut and cook, stirring constantly, until golden brown, 2-3 minutes. Transfer to a plate. Turn off heat and wipe out pan.

Pierce green bean bag with a fork; place bag on a plate. Microwave until tender, 1-2 minutes. (TIP: No microwave? No problem! Steam beans in a small pot with a splash of water until just tender, 6-8 minutes.) Transfer to a medium bowl and toss with 1 TBSP butter until melted. Season with salt and pepper. Keep covered until ready to serve.

Pat tilapia dry with paper towels; season generously with salt and pepper. Rub all over with turmeric. Heat a large drizzle of oil in pan used for coconut over medium-high heat. Add tilapia; cook until firm and cooked through, 4-6 minutes per side. Turn off heat; transfer to a plate. Wipe out pan. Heat a drizzle of oil in same pan over medium heat. Add ginger, shallot, and garlic; cook, stirring, until fragrant, 1 minute. Stir in ¼ cup water (⅓ cup for 4), stock concentrate, and juice from half the lime. Simmer until slightly reduced, 2-3 minutes. Turn off heat.

Add 2 TBSP butter to pan with sauce. Stir in half the cilantro and season with salt and pepper. Fluff rice; stir in 1 TBSP butter, coconut, and lime zest. Divide rice, green beans, and tilapia between plates. Spoon sauce over tilapia. Sprinkle with remaining cilantro. Serve with remaining lime wedges on the side.

Nutrition

Energy (kJ)3012 kJ
Calories720 kcal
Fat39 g
Saturated Fat11 g
Carbohydrate61 g
Sugar10 g
Dietary Fiber5 g
Protein34 g
Cholesterol125 mg
Sodium560 mg

Broiled Salmon Fillets

Prep: 10 mins
Cook: 15 mins
Servings: 4

Ingredients

1 teaspoon sesame seeds
2 tablespoons mirin (Japanese sweet wine)
1 tablespoon soy sauce
1 teaspoon honey
2 tablespoons miso paste
1 tablespoon oil, or as needed
1 pound salmon fillets
1 tablespoon minced ginger

Directions

Toast sesame seeds in a small saucepan over medium heat, stirring occasionally, about 2 minutes. Watch them closely and remove from heat once sesame seeds are a golden brown. Set aside.
Combine miso paste, mirin, soy sauce, ginger, and honey in a small bowl. Mix well. Stir in toasted sesame seeds.
Set an oven rack about 6 inches from the heat source and preheat the oven's broiler. Line a baking pan with foil and lightly grease with oil. Coat salmon well in the miso sauce and place skin-side up on the baking pan.
Broil in the preheated oven, watching closely, until fish flakes easily with a fork, 12 to 15 minutes.

Nutrition

240 calories; protein 25.7g; carbohydrates 6.9g; fat 11g; cholesterol 50.4mg; sodium 595.8mg.

Tilapia Casserole

Prep 10 mins
Cook: 40 mins
Servings: 7

Tilapia Ingredients:

2 lbs (about 6-10 count) Tilapia fillets, thawed
Olive Oil to saute
1 Tbsp mayo
1 Tbsp ketchup

Marinade Ingredients:

2 large eggs
1 cup buttermilk
1/2 tsp Salt and 1/8 teaspoon Pepper
2 Tbsp soy sauce
Vegetable Ingredients:
2 medium bell peppers (red, orange, or yellow)
1 medium onion
2 medium/large carrots, julienned or grated

Directions:

Whisk together marinade ingredients. Combine with tilapia in a large ziploc bag or bowl and marinate in the fridge at least 1 1/2 hours. Slice onions into thin half circles, slice bell pepper into thin strips and julienne or grate carrots. In a large skillet over medium/high, heat 2-3 Tbsp oil and saute onions for 3 minutes or until softened. Add sliced bell peppers and carrots and saute another 5 min or until softened. Remove from pan and set veggies aside.

Once fish is done marinating, drain and discard marinade. In the same empty skillet over medium/high, add 2-3 Tbsp oil and saute fish lightly on the skillet just until golden on the outside (2 min per side) – it's ok if it's not cooked through completely at this point.

Layer the casserole dish with 1/2 of the vegetables on the bottom. Place fish over the vegetables. Stir together 1 Tbsp ketchup and 1 Tbsp mayo and brush this mixture evenly over the top of the fish. Cover fish with remaining veggies. Sprinkle the top with salt and pepper

Oysters Rockefeller

Prep:30 mins
Cook:30 mins
Servings:6

Ingredients

2 slices bacon
1 ½ cups cooked spinach
⅓ cup bread crumbs
¼ cup chopped green onions
1 tablespoon chopped fresh parsley
½ teaspoon salt
24 unopened, fresh, live medium oysters
3 tablespoons extra virgin olive oil
1 teaspoon anise flavored liqueur
4 cups kosher salt
1 dash hot pepper sauce

Directions

Preheat oven to 450 degrees F . Place bacon in a large, deep skillet. Cook over medium high heat until evenly brown. Drain, crumble and set aside.

Clean oysters and place in a large stockpot. Pour in enough water to cover oysters; bring the water and oysters to a boil. Remove from heat and drain and cool oysters. When cooled break the top shell off of each oyster.

Using a food processor, chop the bacon, spinach, bread crumbs, green onions, and parsley. Add the salt, hot sauce, olive oil and anise-flavored liqueur and process until finely chopped but not pureed, about 10 seconds.

Arrange the oysters in their half shells on a pan with kosher salt. Spoon some of the spinach mixture on each oyster. Bake 10 minutes until cooked through, then change the oven's setting to broil and broil until browned on top. Serve hot.

Nutrition

148 calories; protein 9.3g; carbohydrates 7.7g; fat 8.9g; cholesterol 18.9mg; sodium 61097.1mg

Tender Goulash

Prep:15 mins
Cook:2 hrs
Servings:8

Ingredients

⅓ cup vegetable oil
2 tablespoons Hungarian sweet paprika
2 teaspoons salt
½ teaspoon ground black pepper
3 pounds beef stew meat, cut into 1 1/2 inch cubes
3 onions, sliced
1 (6 ounce) can tomato paste
1 clove garlic, minced
1 teaspoon salt
1 ½ cups water

Directions

Heat oil in a large pot or Dutch oven over medium heat. Cook onions
in oil until soft, stirring frequently. Remove onions and set aside.
In a medium bowl, combine paprika, 2 teaspoons salt and pepper.
Coat beef cubes in spice mixture, and cook in onion pot until brown
on all sides. Return the onions to the pot, and pour in tomato paste,
water, garlic and the remaining 1 teaspoon salt. Reduce heat to low,
cover and simmer, stirring occasionally, 1 1/2 to 2 hours, or until meat
is tender.

Nutrition

:
549 calories; protein 32.8g; carbohydrates 9.4g; fat 42.3g; cholesterol
114mg; sodium 1138.5mg.

Honey Fish

Prep:10 mins
Cook:15 mins
Additional:15 mins
Servings:4

Ingredients

1 teaspoon ground ginger
1 teaspoon garlic powder
¼ cup honey
1 green onion, chopped
⅓ cup orange juice
1 (1 1/2-pound) salmon fillet
⅓ cup soy sauce

Directions

In a large self-closing plastic bag, combine ginger, garlic, soy sauce, orange juice, honey, and green onion; mix well. Place salmon in bag and seal tightly. Turn bag gently to distribute marinade. Refrigerate for 20 to 30 minutes.
Preheat an outdoor grill for medium heat and lightly oil grate. Remove salmon from marinade, shake off excess, and discard remaining marinade. Grill for 12 to 15 minutes per inch of thickness, or until the fish flakes easily with a fork.

Nutrition

:
373 calories; protein 37.6g; carbohydrates 22.3g; fat 14.5g; cholesterol 114mg; sodium 1291mg.

Cilantro Beef

Prep/Total Time: 30 min.

Ingredients

1 beef flank steak (1 pound)
1/2 teaspoon salt
4 teaspoons olive oil, divided
1 medium onion, halved and sliced
1/4 teaspoon pepper
1 jalapeno pepper, seeded and finely chopped
1/2 cup salsa
1/4 cup minced fresh cilantro
2 teaspoons lime juice
1 garlic clove, minced
Dash hot pepper sauce
Optional toppings: salsa, cilantro, shredded lettuce and sour cream
8 flour tortillas (6 inches), warmed

Directions

Sprinkle steak with salt and pepper. In a large skillet, heat 2 teaspoons oil over medium-high heat. Add steak; cook 5-7 minutes on each side or until meat reaches desired doneness (for medium-rare, a thermometer should read 135°; medium, 140°; medium-well, 145°). Remove from pan.

In same skillet, heat remaining oil over medium heat. Add onion; cook and stir 4-5 minutes or until tender. Add jalapeno and garlic; cook 2 minutes longer. Stir in salsa, cilantro, lime juice and pepper sauce; heat through.

Thinly slice steak across the grain; stir into onion mixture. Serve in tortillas; top as desired.

Crispy Fish Fillets

Prep:10 mins
Cook:10 mins
Servings:4

Ingredients

1 egg
4 (6 ounce) fillets sole
½ teaspoon salt
1 ½ cups instant mashed potato flakes
¼ cup oil for frying
2 tablespoons prepared yellow mustard

Directions

In a shallow dish, whisk together the egg, mustard, and salt; set aside.
Place the potato flakes in another shallow dish.
Heat oil in a large heavy skillet over medium-high heat.
Dip fish fillets in the egg mixture. Dredge the fillets in the potato flakes, making sure to completely coat the fish. For extra crispy, dip into egg and potato flakes again.
Fry fish fillets in oil for 3 to 4 minutes on each side, or until golden brown.

Nutrition

391 calories; protein 30g; carbohydrates 26.2g; fat 18.1g; cholesterol 136.8mg; sodium 655.9mg.

Cumin Beef

Cook: 15 mins
Prep: 5 mins
Servings: 2

Ingredients

700 g rump Beef
4 teaspoon finely chopped ginger
4 fresh red chilli, seeded, finely chopped
4 spring onions only the green parts, in very fine rings
4-8 teaspoon dried chilli flakes
4 teaspoon ground cumin
2 tablespoons finely chopped garlic
salt
500 ml Plenty of oil for frying
Marinade
2 tablespoons Shaoxing wine
1 sachet of baking powder
2 teaspoon light soy sauce
1 teaspoon salt
2 teaspoon dark soy sauce
2 tablespoons water
2 tablespoons potato starch

DIRECTIONS

Cut meat against the grain into thin slices about 4 cm x 3 cm and then
marinate.
The oil in a wok heat up to around 140 ° C. pour in meat in two
stages, and stir thoroughly. Once the pieces separate from each other,
remove and allow to drain well on the large slotted spoon.

Drain Oil up to 4 tbsp. Then add in strong flame ginger, garlic, fresh chilies, possibly pepper flakes and cumin and stir fry briefly. give meat back into the wok and mix well, season with salt.

When all the ingredients sizzle nice and smell good, the F-onion rings fold briefly take wok from the heat, stir in sesame oil and serve.

Chow Mein

Prep:20 mins
Cook:15 mins
Additional:20 mins
Servings:4

Ingredients

2 teaspoons soy sauce

¼ teaspoon sesame oil

½ pound skinless, boneless chicken breast halves, cut into strips

¾ cup chicken broth

1 teaspoon cornstarch

2 tablespoons oyster sauce

1 carrot, cut into thin strips

½ pound chow mein noodles

1 teaspoon minced garlic

2 heads bok choy, chopped

½ zucchini, diced

¾ teaspoon white sugar

1 tablespoon vegetable oil

10 sugar snap peas

2 tablespoons chopped green onion

Directions

Whisk soy sauce, corn starch, and sesame oil together in a large bowl until smooth; add chicken strips and toss to coat. Cover and refrigerate for at least 20 minutes.

Combine chicken broth, oyster sauce, and sugar in a small bowl and set aside.

Bring a large pot of water to a boil. Add noodles and cook over medium heat until cooked through but still firm to the bite, 4 to 6 minutes. Drain and rinse with cold water.

Heat vegetable oil in a large skillet. Cook and garlic in hot oil for 30 seconds; add marinated chicken. Cook and stir until browned and no longer pink in the center, 5 to 6 minutes. Remove chicken mixture to a plate. Cook and stir bok choy, zucchini, snap peas, and carrot in the hot skillet until softened, about 2 minutes. Return noodles and chicken mixture to the skillet. Pour broth mixture into noodle mixture; cook and stir until warmed through, about 2 minutes. Serve garnished with green onions.

Nutrition

527 calories; protein 29.4g; carbohydrates 61.7g; fat 17.9g; cholesterol 30.2mg; sodium 991.7mg.

Curry Beef

Servings:6

Ingredients

2 tablespoons butter
1 pound cubed beef stew meat
6 cups beef stock
2 tablespoons curry powder
2 onions, chopped
2 bay leaves
2 tablespoons distilled white vinegar
2 teaspoons salt
2 potatoes, sliced

Directions

Melt the butter in a large saucepan. Cook onions and beef cubes until beef is browned and onions are tender.
Add the beef stock, curry and bay leaves. Cook over low heat for 30 minutes.
Add the potatoes, vinegar and salt. Simmer for 45 minutes to 1 hour until all is tender. Remove bay leaves, and serve hot.

Nutrition

343 calories; protein 20g; carbohydrates 20.5g; fat 19.8g; cholesterol 60.8mg; sodium 939.2mg.

Steak Soup

Prep:45 mins

Cook:1 hr 30 mins

Servings:8

Ingredients

2 tablespoons vegetable oil

1 ½ pounds lean boneless beef round steak, cut into cubes

½ cup chopped onion

3 tablespoons all-purpose flour

1 tablespoon paprika

2 tablespoons butter

1 teaspoon salt

4 cups beef broth

2 cups water

4 sprigs fresh parsley, chopped

¼ teaspoon ground black pepper

2 tablespoons chopped celery leaves

1 bay leaf

½ teaspoon dried marjoram

1 ½ cups sliced carrots

1 ½ cups chopped celery

1 (6 ounce) can tomato paste

1 ½ cups peeled, diced Yukon Gold potatoes

1 (15.25 ounce) can whole kernel corn, drained

Directions

Melt butter and oil in a large skillet over medium heat until the foam disappears from the butter, and stir in the steak cubes and onion. Cook and stir until the meat and onion are browned, about 10 minutes. While beef is cooking, mix together flour, paprika, salt, and pepper in a bowl. Sprinkle the flour mixture over the browned meat, and stir to coat.

In a large soup pot, pour in the beef broth and water, and stir in the parsley, celery leaves, bay leaf, and marjoram. Stir in beef mixture, and bring to a boil. Reduce heat to medium-low, cover the pot, and simmer, stirring occasionally, until meat is tender, about 45 minutes. Mix in the potatoes, carrots, celery, tomato paste, and corn; bring the soup back to a simmer, and cook uncovered, stirring occasionally, until the vegetables are tender and the soup is thick, 15 to 20 minutes. Remove bay leaf and serve hot.

Nutrition

361 calories; protein 36g; carbohydrates 26.9g; fat 12.9g; cholesterol 84.1mg; sodium 1118.2mg.

Bream with Fennel

Prep Time10 minutes
Cook Time50 minutes
Servings4 people

Ingredients

2 tablespoons olive oil
1 small fennel bulb finely sliced
1 garlic clove crushed or very finely chopped
2 large baking potatoes peeled and finely sliced
1 small onion finely sliced
100 ml white wine
2 whole sea bream gutted (get your fishmonger to do this)
½ lemon zested then sliced
Salt and pepper (to taste)
2 sprigs thyme
2 sprigs parsley
Small handful of parsley chopped
2 sprigs rosemary

Directions

Preheat your oven to 200C /180C fan / gas mark 6 / 400F.
Place the fennel, onions, potatoes and garlic in a large roasting tray. (It should be big enough to fit the fish comfortably.)
Pour over the oil and add salt and pepper to taste, then turn the veggies over in the oil so everything gets coated evenly. Spread the vegetables out over the base of the tray.
Pour in the white wine – but pour the wine carefully down the side so it doesn't wash off the olive oil that you've just coated the veggies with.

Cover the dish tightly with foil and bake for 20 minutes, then uncover and bake for a further 10 minutes.

Now season the fish and stuff with slices of lemon and sprigs of thyme, rosemary and parsley. Pop your fish on top of the vegetables and cook uncovered for a further 20 minutes.

Finely chop the remaining parsley and mix with the lemon zest. Scatter over the fish and voilà - gorgeous looking food, very little faff.

Wonton Soup

Prep:30 mins
Cook:5 mins
Additional:40 mins
Servings:8

Ingredients

½ pound boneless pork loin, coarsely chopped
1 teaspoon brown sugar
1 tablespoon Chinese rice wine
1 tablespoon light soy sauce
1 teaspoon finely chopped green onion
2 ounces peeled shrimp, finely chopped
24 (3.5 inch square) wonton wrappers
3 cups chicken stock
1 teaspoon chopped fresh ginger root
⅛ cup finely chopped green onion

Directions

In a large bowl, combine pork, shrimp, sugar, wine, soy sauce, 1
teaspoon chopped green onion and ginger. Blend well, and let stand
for 25 to 30 minutes.
Place about one teaspoon of the filling at the center of each wonton
skin. Moisten all 4 edges of wonton wrapper with water, then pull the
top corner down to the bottom, folding the wrapper over the filling to
make a triangle. Press edges firmly to make a seal. Bring left and right
corners together above the filling. Overlap the tips of these corners,
moisten with water and press together. Continue until all wrappers are
used.

FOR SOUP: Bring the chicken stock to a rolling boil. Drop wontons in, and cook for 5 minutes. Garnish with chopped green onion, and serve.

Nutrition

145 calories; protein 9.9g; carbohydrates 15.3g; fat 4.2g; cholesterol 32.5mg; sodium 588.8mg

Shrimp and Catfish Gumbo

Prep:30 mins
Cook:1 hr
Servings:10

Ingredients

¼ cup cooking oil
1 bell pepper, chopped
2 cloves garlic, minced
1 large onion, chopped
4 cubes beef bouillon
2 stalks celery, chopped
1 (16 ounce) package frozen sliced okra
4 cups shrimp, peeled and deveined
6 cups hot water
1 (28 ounce) can diced tomatoes, undrained
¼ teaspoon cayenne pepper
½ teaspoon dried thyme
2 teaspoons salt
2 bay leaves
2 pounds catfish fillets, cut into 1 inch pieces
1 teaspoon dry crab boil

Directions

Warm oil in a skillet over medium heat. Stir in onion, bell pepper,
celery, and garlic. Cook until soft, about 10 minutes.
Dissolve bouillon cubes in hot water. Pour into skillet. Stir tomatoes,
okra, and shrimp into skillet. Season with salt, cayenne pepper, thyme,
bay leaves, and crab boil. Bring to a boil; cover, and simmer 30
minutes.

Place fish in skillet, return to boil; cover, and simmer 15 minutes more. Remove bay leaves, and serve.

Nutrition

269 calories; protein 26.5g; carbohydrates 8.8g; fat 13.5g; cholesterol 120.6mg; sodium 1030mg.

Thai Tofu Soup

Prep:25 mins
Cook:15 mins
Servings:4

Ingredients

1 onion, chopped
2 tablespoons Thai red curry paste
1 tablespoon grated ginger
1 tablespoon grated garlic
1 tablespoon vegetable oil
1 (14 ounce) can coconut milk
1 tablespoon white sugar
1 pinch salt and ground black pepper to taste
1 (32 fluid ounce) container vegetable broth
1 (12 ounce) package extra-firm tofu, cut into small cubes
4 ounces cauliflower florets, cut into bite-sized pieces
4 ounces mushrooms, cut into bite-size pieces
4 ounces broccoli, chopped into bite-sized pieces

Directions

Heat oil in a large pot over medium heat. Add onion, curry paste,
ginger, and garlic. Stir continuously until onion begins to soften, about
2 minutes. Pour in vegetable broth and coconut milk. Add sugar. Bring
to a boil. Stir in tofu, broccoli, cauliflower, and mushrooms.
Reduce heat and cover pot. Simmer soup, stirring occasionally, until
vegetables are tender, 6 to 8 minutes. Season with salt and pepper.

Onion Beef Gravy

Prep:5 mins
Cook:36 mins
Servings:8

Ingredients

cooking spray
1 (1 ounce) package dry onion soup mix
1 teaspoon beef base (such as Better Than Bouillon®)
1 teaspoon minced garlic
3 cups water
3 tablespoons all-purpose flour
¼ cup milk
ground black pepper to taste

Directions

Spray a saucepan with cooking spray. Add garlic and cook over medium heat just until fragrant, about 1 minute. Add water, onion soup mix, and beef base; bring to a boil. Cover the pan and simmer until onions are tender, about 20 minutes.
Combine milk and flour in a jar with a lid; shake until combined and whisk into the saucepan. Bring gravy back to a boil and cook until thickened, about 10 minutes. Season with black pepper.

Nutrition

26 calories; protein 0.9g; carbohydrates 5.1g; fat 0.3g; cholesterol 0.6mg; sodium 370.4mg

Chicory Soup

Servings: 6
Cook: 10 mins
Prep: 5 mins

Ingredients

Serves 4-6 people
2 heads of chicory
200g (7 oz) of rice
Olive oil, preferably of the dark green 'fruity' kind
Salt and pepper
2-3 cloves of garlic, peeled and slightly crushed

Directions

You trim and cut up the chicory (or just the green parts—see Notes below) into smallish pieces, throw it into some well salted boiling water and cook for about 5 minutes or so.
You then transfer the chicory (use a slotted spoon, as you'll need the "broth" for later) into a pan in which you will have sautéed the garlic in olive oil. Let the chicory insaporire—absorb the flavors of the seasoned oil—for a minute or two, then add a few ladlefuls of the chicory 'broth' until you have the quantity of soup you like.
Add rice and allow to simmer until the rice and chicory are tender. (If you have some cooked rice on hand, just add it at the very end, as when I made this soup, using some leftover white rice from a Chinese restaurant).
Serve your chicory and rice soup in deep plates and top with pecorino cheese, freshly ground pepper and un filo d'olio–a drizzle of olive oil.

Tarragon Beef Stew

Prep:15 mins
Cook:3 hrs
Servings:6

Ingredients

1 pound beef stew meat
6 cups chicken broth
¼ teaspoon pepper
2 tablespoons butter
4 cups water
2 cups new potatoes
2 large carrots, quartered
4 cloves garlic
1 ½ cups sweet vermouth
2 teaspoons chopped fresh tarragon
½ cup Worcestershire sauce
1 tablespoon white sugar
1 tablespoon honey
 bay leaf
¼ teaspoon salt

Directions

Melt butter In a large stockpot over medium-high heat. Add the beef
stew meat, and fry for 2 to 3 minutes, or until evenly browned on the
outside.
Pour the chicken broth, water, and vermouth into the stock pot. Add
the potatoes, carrots, and garlic. Season with tarragon, bay leaf,
Worcestershire sauce, sugar, honey, salt and pepper. Bring to a boil,
reduce heat, and cover. Cook 2 1/2 hours to blend the flavors.

Remove cover and continue cooking 20 minutes, or long enough to evaporate enough liquid to reach your desired thickness.

Nutrition

450 calories; protein 21.2g; carbohydrates 29.7g; fat 20.2g; cholesterol 76.6mg; sodium 423.5mg.

Soup of onion

Prep:15 mins
Cook:1 hr
Servings:4

Ingredients

1 teaspoon salt
2 large red onions, thinly sliced
2 large sweet onions, thinly sliced
4 tablespoons butter
1 (48 fluid ounce) can chicken broth
½ cup red wine
1 tablespoon Worcestershire sauce
1 (14 ounce) can beef broth
2 sprigs fresh parsley
1 bay leaf
1 tablespoon balsamic vinegar
1 sprig fresh thyme leaves
salt and freshly ground black pepper to taste
8 slices Gruyere or Swiss cheese slices, room temperature
½ cup shredded Asiago or mozzarella cheese, room temperature
4 thick slices French or Italian bread
4 pinches paprika

Directions

Melt butter in a large pot over medium-high heat. Stir in salt, red
onions and sweet onions. Cook 35 minutes, stirring frequently, until
onions are caramelized and almost syrupy.
Mix chicken broth, beef broth, red wine and Worcestershire sauce into
pot. Bundle the parsley, thyme, and bay leaf with twine and place in
pot. Simmer over medium heat for 20 minutes, stirring occasionally.

Remove and discard the herbs. Reduce the heat to low, mix in vinegar and season with salt and pepper. Cover and keep over low heat to stay hot while you prepare the bread.

Preheat oven broiler. Arrange bread slices on a baking sheet and broil 3 minutes, turning once, until well toasted on both sides. Remove from heat; do not turn off broiler.

Arrange 4 large oven safe bowls or crocks on a rimmed baking sheet. Fill each bowl 2/3 full with hot soup. Top each bowl with 1 slice toasted bread, 2 slice Gruyere cheese and 1/4 of the Asiago or mozzarella cheese. Sprinkle a little bit of paprika over the top of each one.

Broil 5 minutes, or until bubbly and golden brown. As it softens, the cheese will cascade over the sides of the crock and form a beautifully melted crusty seal. Serve immediately!

Nutrition

618 calories; protein 29.7g; carbohydrates 39.5g; fat 35.9g; cholesterol 113.9mg; sodium 335.7mg

Sorrel Soup

Prep:10 mins
Cook:10 mins
Servings:6

Ingredients

2 tablespoons uncooked white rice
salt and pepper to taste
1 bunch sorrel, stemmed and rinsed
½ cup heavy cream
3 cups vegetable broth

Directions

In a large saucepan, bring broth to a boil over medium-high heat. Stir in rice, reduce heat, and simmer for about 8 minutes. Stir in sorrel and return to a boil. Remove from heat and puree in batches in a blender or food processor or using an immersion blender.
Return to medium-low heat and stir in cream, salt, and pepper. Heat through and serve.

Nutrition

112 calories; protein 1.5g; carbohydrates 9.5g; fat 7.8g; cholesterol 27.2mg; sodium 239.3mg.

Carrot Meatballs

Serves 4
Cook: 45 minutes

INGREDIENTS

1 pound ground beef
½ teaspoon black pepper
1 medium yellow onion, minced
2 teaspoons garlic, minced
1 large carrot, grated
1 tablespoon tomato paste
1 teaspoon salt
1 tablespoon dried Italian seasoning

Directions

Preheat oven to 350°F. Lightly grease a baking sheet with cooking spray.
Mix beef, carrot, onion, garlic, Italian seasoning, tomato paste, salt, and pepper, with a fork or with clean hands, until well combined.
Roll into meatballs, roughly one heaping tablespoon in size. Space meatballs apart for even cooking. Bake for 25 minutes.
Remove from oven to rest for 5 minutes before serving.

CHAPTER 4: **SNACKS AND SIDES RECIPES**

Cinnamon Chips

Prep:5 mins
Cook: 35 mins
Servings: 24

Ingredients

⅓ cup white sugar
1 tablespoon light corn syrup
2 teaspoons ground cinnamon
1 tablespoon vegetable shortening

Directions

Stir sugar, ground cinnamon, shortening, and corn syrup together in a small bowl until dough comes together. Place dough between two layers of parchment paper; roll to 1/8- to 1/4-inch thick. Transfer to a baking sheet; remove top piece of parchment paper.
Bake in preheated oven until golden and bubbly, about 35 minutes.
Cool completely and break into pieces.

Nutrition

18 calories; carbohydrates 3.6g; fat 0.5g; sodium 0.5mg.

Tuna and Hummus on Flatbread

Ingredients

1 7 ounce Bumble Bee Albacore tuna in oil
1/2 tsp. Dijon mustard
2 Tbsp. minced celery
1/2 Tbsp. diced green onion
radished sliced
1 Tbsp. minced cornichons aka mini gherkin pickles
1 Tbsp. mayonnaise
1 Tbsp. reserved oil from tuna
1 Tbsp. fresh lemon juice
1/4 tsp. salt
1/8 tsp. pepper
your favorite bread
hummus
1/4 cup cannellini beans

Directions

Drain the oil from the tuna, reserving the oil. Place the tuna in a mixing bowl and flake it with a fork.

Add the celery, onion, cornichons, lemon juice, mayo, 1 tablespoon of the reserved oil, mustard, salt, and pepper and mix well. Add in cannellini beans and stir.

(Can cover and refrigerate for a few hours to allow the flavors to develop or go ahead and make the sandwiches if needed.)

Spread bread slices with a layer of hummus. Spread the tuna mixture on each piece of bread. Top with slices of radish, and serve immediately.

Jalapeno Crisp

YIELDS:8 CUPS
PREP TIME:0 HOURS 15 MINS
COOK TIME:0 HOURS 10 MINS
TOTAL TIME:0 HOURS 25 MINS

INGREDIENTS

4 slices bacon
1 c. finely shredded Parmesan
1/2 c. shredded cheddar (preferably aged)
1 jalapeño, sliced thinly
Freshly ground black pepper

DIRECTIONS

Preheat oven to 375°. In a large nonstick skillet over medium
heat, cook bacon until crispy, 8 minutes. Drain on a paper towel-lined
plate, then chop.
Spoon about 1 tablespoon of Parmesan into a small mound on a large
baking sheet and top with about tablespoon of cheddar cheese.
Carefully pat down cheeses and top with a jalapeño slice. Sprinkle with
bacon and season with pepper. Repeat with remaining ingredients.
Bake until crispy and golden, about 12 minutes.
Let cool slightly on pan before serving.

Potatoes Croquettes

Prep:10 mins
Cook:10 mins
Servings:4

Ingredients

4 cups mashed potatoes
2 tablespoons dried parsley
½ cup grated Romano cheese
salt and pepper to taste
2 eggs
1 teaspoon dried onion flakes
1 cup Italian-style dried bread crumbs
1 quart vegetable oil for deep frying
2 tablespoons imitation bacon bits

Directions

In a large bowl, combine mashed potatoes, eggs, parsley, cheese, salt and pepper, bacon bits and onion flakes. Form mixture into patties, and dredge patties in the bread crumbs.
Pour oil 1/2 inch deep in a large, heavy skillet. Heat oil over medium-high heat. Fry patties, flipping to fry them on both sides, until they are golden brown. Serve hot.

Nutrition

660 calories; protein 17.6g; carbohydrates 58.4g; fat 39.9g; cholesterol 110.9mg; sodium 1505.6mg.

Mixes of Snack

Prep:10 mins
Cook:17 mins
Servings:16

Ingredients

Cooking spray
1 cup untoasted walnut halves
½ cup white sugar
1 cup untoasted pecan halves
1 cup unsalted, dry roasted cashews
1 teaspoon salt
½ teaspoon freshly ground black pepper
¼ teaspoon ground cumin
1 cup unsalted, dry roasted almonds
¼ teaspoon cayenne pepper
¼ cup water
1 tablespoon butter

Directions

Preheat oven to 350 degrees F. Line a baking sheet with aluminum foil and lightly coat with cooking spray.
Combine walnut halves, pecan halves, almonds, and cashews in a large bowl. Add salt, black pepper, cumin, and cayenne pepper; toss to coat. Heat sugar, water, and butter in a small saucepan over medium heat until the butter is melted. Cook for 1 minute and remove from heat. Slowly pour butter mixture over the bowl of nuts and stir to coat. Transfer nuts to the prepared baking sheet and spread into a single layer.

Bake nuts in the preheated oven for 10 minutes. Stir nuts until the warm syrup coats every nut. Spread into a single layer, return to the oven, and bake until nuts are sticky and roasted, about 6 minutes. Allow to cool before serving.

Nutrition

219 calories; protein 4.8g; carbohydrates 12.7g; fat 18.1g; cholesterol 1.9mg; sodium 205.7mg.

Kale Popcorn

PREP TIME5 minutes
COOK TIME15 minutes
MAKES8 cups

Ingredients

Kale Dust
1 bundle of Lacinato kale (aka dinosaur or Tuscan) (usually 9 to 10
ounces or 255 to 285 grams; if using curly kale, go for a 1-pound
(454g) bunch))
1 tablespoon (15 ml) olive oil
Fine sea salt
Popcorn
4 to 5 tablespoons (60 to 75 ml) olive oil
1/3 cup (70 grams) popcorn kernels
2/3 cup (95 grams) finely grated Pecorino Romano
Fine sea salt and freshly ground black pepper, to taste

Directions

Kale Dust
Heat the oven to 300°F. Rinse and dry the kale; no worries if you
don't get every last droplet of water off. Remove and discard the tough
stems.
Lightly brush two large baking sheets with olive oil—the thinnest coat
is just fine. Arrange the leaves in one layer on the prepared baking
sheet(s), sprinkle lightly with salt, and bake for 12 to 14 minutes, until
the leaves are crisp. Let cool completely. In a food processor, with a
mortar and pestle, or even with a muddler in a bowl, grind the kale
chips down into a coarse powder.
Popcorn

Place 3 tablespoons of olive oil and 2 or 3 kernels of popcorn in a 3-quart or larger pot. Turn the heat to medium-high, and cover with a lid. When you hear these first kernels pop, add the remaining kernels and replace the lid. Using pot holders, shimmy the pot around to keep the kernels moving as they pop. When several seconds pass between pops, remove the pot from the heat.

Transfer the popcorn to a bowl, and immediately toss with the remaining 1 to 2 tablespoons olive oil, kale dust, Pecorino, salt, and a few grinds of black pepper. Toss until evenly coated. Taste, and adjust the seasonings if needed.

Egg White Sandwich

10 minPrep Time
20 minCook Time
30 minTotal Time

Ingredients

4 Bagel Thins (I used Everything Bagel Thins)
8 egg whites
1 tomato (sliced)
1 avocado (sliced)
1 cup spinach
4 Tablespoons tomatillo salsa
4 mozzarella cheese slices

Directions

Toast bagel thins.
In a small skillet over medium heat, cook egg whites (almost like you would cook a fried egg - I cooked them two egg whites at a time). Top the bottom half of each bagel thin with an equal amount of spinach, egg whites, tomato slices, avocado slices, mozzarella cheese, tomatillo salsa. Top with the other half of the bagel thin.

Peas Hummus

Total Time: 5 minutes
Servings: 10

Ingredients

400 g (15 oz) can of chickpeas - not yet drained (garbanzo beans)
Pinch of salt and pepper
150 g (1 cup) fresh or frozen peas
2 tsp lemon juice
1 clove of garlic minced
2 tbsp tahini

Directions

Drain the chickpeas over a bowl to collect the liquid (aquafaba), then
add the chickpeas to a blender or food processor.
Run the frozen peas under hot water to thaw, then also add them to
the blender, along with the tahini, lemon juice, garlic salt and pepper as
well as 4 tbsp of the aquafaba.
Blend for a few minutes until thick and creamy. You may need to
scrape the sides down periodically. Add a little more aquafaba if
necessary to get it a thick and creamy consistency.

Nutrition

Calories: 63kcal Carbohydrates: 8g Protein: 3g Fat: 2g Sodium: 3mg Po
tassium: 108mg Fiber: 2g Sugar: 1g Vitamin A: 120IU Vitamin
C: 6.8mg Calcium: 18mg Iron: 0.9mg

Baked Olives

Prep:25 mins
Cook:15 mins
Servings:12

Ingredients

3 ½ cups whole mixed olives, drained
2 tablespoons fresh orange juice
2 tablespoons olive oil
¼ teaspoon crushed red pepper flakes
2 cloves garlic, minced
¼ cup dry white wine
2 tablespoons fresh parsley, chopped
1 ½ tablespoons chopped fresh oregano
 sprigs fresh rosemary
4 teaspoons grated orange zest

Directions

Preheat oven to 375 degrees F. Stir the olives together with the wine, orange juice, olive oil, and garlic in a 9x13 inch baking dish. Nestle the sprigs of rosemary in the olives.
Bake in the preheated oven for 15 minutes, stirring halfway through the baking. Remove and discard the rosemary sprigs, then stir in the parsley, oregano, orange zest, and red pepper flakes. Serve warm, or cool the olives and use them to top a salad.

Nutrition

75 calories; protein 0.7g; carbohydrates 1.4g; fat 7.5g; sodium 980.9mg

Broccoli Nuggets

Prep:15 mins
Cook:25 mins
Servings:4

Ingredients

1 teaspoon vegetable oil, or as needed
1 cup bread crumbs
1 ½ cups shredded Cheddar cheese
3 eggs
½ teaspoon dried basil
1 (16 ounce) package frozen chopped broccoli, thawed
½ teaspoon dried oregano
¼ teaspoon garlic powder

Directions

Preheat oven to 375 degrees F . Grease a baking sheet with oil.
Place a steamer insert into a saucepan and fill with water to just below
the bottom of the steamer. Bring water to a boil; add broccoli, cover,
and steam until tender, 3 to 6 minutes. Let broccoli cool at room
temperature until cool enough to touch.
Transfer broccoli into a large mixing bowl. Add bread crumbs,
Cheddar cheese, eggs, basil, oregano, and garlic powder to the
broccoli; mix. Shape into nuggets or fun shapes and arrange onto the
prepared baking sheet.
Bake in preheated for 15 minutes, flip, and continue baking until
heated through and beginning to firm, 12 to 15 minutes more.

Nutrition

372 calories; protein 22.1g; carbohydrates 26.1g; fat 20.7g; cholesterol 184mg; sodium 540.7mg.

Baked Zucchini Chips

Prep:5 mins
Cook:10 mins
Servings:4

Ingredients

2 medium zucchini, cut into 1/4-inch slices
½ cup seasoned dry bread crumbs
2 tablespoons grated Parmesan cheese
2 egg whites
⅛ teaspoon ground black pepper

Directions

Preheat the oven to 475 degrees F.
In one small bowl, stir together the bread crumbs, pepper and
Parmesan cheese. Place the egg whites in a separate bowl. Dip zucchini
slices into the egg whites, then coat the breadcrumb mixture. Place on
a greased baking sheet.
Bake for 5 minutes in the preheated oven, then turn over and bake for
another 6 to 10 minutes, until browned and crispy.

Nutrition

92 calories; protein 6.1g; carbohydrates 13.8g; fat 1.7g; cholesterol
2.4mg; sodium 339.6mg.

Onion Dip

Total:5 mins

Servings:6

Ingredients

¼ cup mayonnaise

1 tablespoon soy sauce

1 tablespoon minced onion

1 ½ teaspoons water, or more as needed

1 tablespoon distilled white vinegar

Directions

Stir the mayonnaise, white vinegar, soy sauce, and water together in a bowl just until combined. Add more water as desired for thinner consistency. Stir in minced onion.

Cover with plastic wrap and refrigerate until cold.

Nutrition

68 calories; protein 0.3g; carbohydrates 0.6g; fat 7.3g; cholesterol 3.5mg; sodium 202.5mg.

Pecan Caramel Corn

yield: 30 SERVINGS
prep time: 30 MINUTES
cook time: 2 HOURS
additional time: 30 MINUTES

INGREDIENTS

15-18 cups popcorn
3/4 teaspoon baking soda
2 cups raw whole pecans
1 1/2 cups brown sugar
1/2 cup light corn syrup
1/4 teaspoon salt
3/4 cups salted butter

DIRECTIONS

Preheat oven to 225 degrees.

Prepare 15-18 cups of plain popcorn. Place popcorn in a large roasting pan and sprinkle 2 cups of raw whole pecans on top of the popcorn.

Heat salted butter, brown sugar, light corn syrup, and salt in a medium heavy saucepan over medium heat. Stir continually with a wooden spoon until the ingredients are melted and well-combined.

Once bubbles begin forming around the edges, cook over medium heat for 5 minutes, without stirring.

Remove from heat and add 3/4 teaspoon of baking soda. Stir until foamy.

Pour the foaming caramel sauce over the prepared popcorn and nuts and stir together until the popcorn and nuts are evenly coated with caramel.

Spread evenly in the roasting pan and bake for 2 hours in the heated oven, stirring every 20 minutes.

Turn over onto wax paper and allow to cool completely, for about 30 minutes.

Store in an airtight containter for up to 3 weeks.

Nutrition Information

Yield30Serving Size1Amount Calories535Total Fat34gSaturated Fat8gTrans Fat7gUnsaturated Fat22gCholesterol12mgSodium635mgCarbohydrates53gFiber8gSugar1 4gProtein6g

Soft Pretzels

Prep:2 hrs
Cook:10 mins
Additional:10 mins
Servings:12

Ingredients

4 teaspoons active dry yeast

1 ¼ cups warm water (110 degrees F)

5 cups all-purpose flour

½ cup white sugar

¼ cup kosher salt, for topping

1 teaspoon white sugar

1 ½ teaspoons salt

½ cup baking soda

4 cups hot water

1 tablespoon vegetable oil

Directions

In a small bowl, dissolve yeast and 1 teaspoon sugar in 1 1/4 cup warm water. Let stand until creamy, about 10 minutes.
In a large bowl, mix together flour, 1/2 cup sugar, and salt. Make a well in the center; add the oil and yeast mixture. Mix and form into a dough. If the mixture is dry, add one or two more tablespoons of water. Knead the dough until smooth, about 6 to 8 minutes. Lightly oil a large bowl, place the dough in the bowl, and turn to coat with oil. Cover with plastic wrap and let rise in a warm place until doubled in size, about 1 hour.
Preheat oven to 450 degrees F. Grease 2 baking sheets.
In a large bowl, dissolve baking soda in 4 cups hot water; set aside.
When risen, turn dough out onto a lightly floured surface and divide

into 12 equal pieces. Roll each piece into a rope and twist into a pretzel shape. Once all of the dough is shaped, dip each pretzel into the baking soda-hot water solution and place pretzels on baking sheets. Sprinkle with kosher salt.

Bake in preheated oven until browned, about 8 minutes.

Nutrition

237 calories; protein 5.9g; carbohydrates 48.9g; fat 1.7g; sodium 4681.1mg.

Mozzarella Cheese Cookies

Prep: 15 mins
Cook: 20 Mins
Servings: 4

INGREDIENTS

- 175g salted butter
- 175g Mozzarella cheese - grated
- 2 egg yolks
- 250g plain flour

DIRECTIONS

Add flour in a mixing bowl.

Remove butter from refrigerator and cut into small cubes.

Rub in the butter with your fingertips until the mixture resembles bread crumbs.

Add egg yolks and grated cheese. Mix with hands until a dough is formed.

Roll out the dough until it's about 5mm in thickness. Cut out the cookies with a cookie cutter.

Place about 2cm apart on a lined baking tray. Brush with egg wash.

Bake in preheated oven at 200 for 18-20 minutes, or till golden in color.

Potato Wedges

Prep:10 mins
Cook:35 mins
Servings:2

Ingredients

2 Russet potatoes, each cut into 6 equal wedges
1 tablespoon herbes de Provence
1 pinch paprika, or to taste
salt and ground black pepper to taste
olive oil

Directions

Preheat oven to 425 degrees F. Line a baking sheet with a silicone baking mat.
Toss potato wedges, olive oil, herbes de Provence, paprika, salt, and black pepper together in a bowl until potatoes are evenly coated. Place wedges on their sides onto the prepared baking sheet.
Bake in the preheated oven for 15 minutes. Flip potatoes onto their other sides; return to oven and cook until crusty and golden brown, about 20 minutes more.

Nutrition

225 calories; protein 4.4g; carbohydrates 37.5g; fat 7g; sodium 13.1mg.

Parmesan Zucchini Rounds

Cook Time: 15 minutes
Total Time: 20 minutes
Servings: 2 to 4 servings

INGREDIENTS

1/2 cup freshly grated Parmesan cheese
2 medium-sized zucchini

Directions

Place oven rack in center position of oven. Preheat to 425°F. Line a
baking sheet with foil (lightly misted with cooking spray
Wash and dry zucchini, and cut into 1/4-inch thick slices. Arrange
zucchini rounds on prepared pan, with little to no space between
them. If desired, lightly sprinkle zucchini with garlic salt and freshly
ground black pepper. Use a small spoon to spread a thin layer of
Parmesan cheese on each slice of zucchini. Bake for 15 to 20 minutes,
or until Parmesan turns a light golden brown. (Watch these closely the
first time you make them and pull them out of the oven early if the
Parmesan is golden before 15 minutes!) Serve immediately.

Nutrition

Calories: 141kcal | Carbohydrates: 7g | Protein: 11g | Fat: 7g | Satura
ted
Fat: 4g | Cholesterol: 22mg | Sodium: 397mg | Potassium: 542mg | F
iber: 1g | Sugar: 5g | Vitamin A: 610IU | Vitamin
C: 35.1mg | Calcium: 309mg | Iron: 1mg

Fresh Tomato Vinaigrette

Prep Time10 mins
Servings: 8

Ingredients

1 fresh red tomato – chopped
1/4 teaspoon pepper
3/4 cup olive oil
1 clove garlic - chopped
1 teaspoon dried oregano
1/2 teaspoon salt
1/4 cup apple cider vinegar

Directions

Add all ingredients to blender, food processor or use a jar and an immersion blender.
Blend until smooth and no large chunks of garlic or tomato remain
Store in a container with a tight fitting lid for up to 5 days in the refrigerator.
(It may separate during this time - just give it a couple shakes).

Nutrition

Fresh Tomato Vinaigrette
Amount Per Serving
Calories 181Calories from Fat 180
% Daily Value*
Fat 20g31%
Saturated Fat 2g10%
Sodium 146mg6%
Potassium 5mg0%

Raspberry Vinaigrette Sauce

PREP TIME: 5 mins
TOTAL TIME: 5 mins
SERVINGS: 12 servings

INGREDIENTS

1 1/2 cups raspberries, fresh or frozen
1/4 cup red wine vinegar
1 small shallot, diced (about 2 tbsp)
1/2 cup olive oil
1/4 tsp salt
1 tsp Dijon mustard
pepper, to taste

DIRECTIONS

Add all ingredients to a food processor and blend for 30 seconds.

NUTRITION

CALORIES: 90kcal, CARBOHYDRATES: 2g, FAT: 9g, SATURATE
D
FAT: 1g, SODIUM: 54mg, POTASSIUM: 29mg, FIBER: 1g, VITAMI
N A: 5iu, VITAMIN C: 4.1mg, CALCIUM: 4mg, IRON: 0.2mg

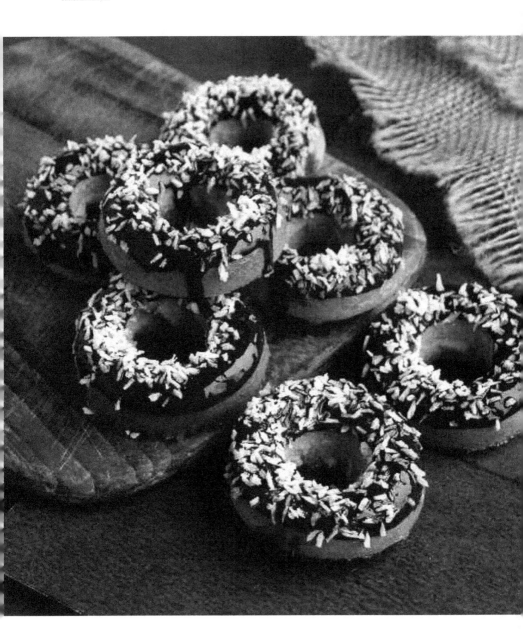

CHAPTER 5: DESSERTS

Chocolate Cake

Servings:12

Ingredients

1 (18.25 ounce) package devil's food cake mix
½ cup warm water
1 (5.9 ounce) package instant chocolate pudding mix
1 cup vegetable oil
4 eggs
1 cup sour cream
2 cups semisweet chocolate chips

Directions

Preheat oven to 350 degrees F.
In a large bowl, mix together the cake and pudding mixes, sour cream, oil, beaten eggs and water. Stir in the chocolate chips and pour batter into a well greased 12 cup bundt pan.
Bake for 50 to 55 minutes, or until top is springy to the touch and a wooden toothpick inserted comes out clean. Cool cake thoroughly in pan at least an hour and a half before inverting onto a plate If desired, dust the cake with powdered sugar.

Nutrition

600 calories; protein 7.6g; carbohydrates 60.9g; fat 38.6g; cholesterol 78.9mg; sodium 550.4mg.

Chocolate Muffins

Servings: 12 muffins
Cook Time: 20 Minutes
Prep: 20 Minutes

INGREDIENTS

2 large eggs
1 cup low fat buttermilk
1 stick (1/2 cup) unsalted butter, melted and slightly cooled
1-3/4 cups all-purpose flour, spooned into measuring cup and leveled-off
2/3 cup natural unsweetened cocoa powder, such as Hershey's
2 teaspoons vanilla extract
1-1/4 cups light brown sugar, packed (be sure it is fresh with no hard lumps)
1 teaspoon baking soda
1/2 teaspoon salt
1 teaspoon baking powder
1cup semi-sweet or bittersweet chocolate chips

DIRECTIONS

Position a rack in the center of the oven and preheat to 425°F. Line a standard 12-cup muffin pan with paper liners.
In a large measuring cup or bowl, whisk together the eggs, buttermilk, and vanilla extract.
In another large bowl, whisk together the flour, cocoa powder, brown sugar, baking powder, baking soda, and salt. Rub the mixture through your fingers to break up any lumps of brown sugar.
To the dry ingredients, add 3/4 cup of the chocolate chips, the buttermilk-egg mixture, and the melted butter. Using a rubber spatula or wooden spoon, mix until until just combined.

Using an ice cream scoop or two spoons, fill the muffin cups to the brim with batter. Distribute the remaining 1/4 cup of chocolate chips evenly over the muffin tops, pressing them lightly into the batter. Place in the oven and bake for 8 minutes, then turn the oven down to 350°F and bake for about 12 minutes more, or until a toothpick inserted in the center of a muffin comes out clean (check a few spots as the melted chocolate chips will make the tester look wet). Transfer to a wire rack and let cool for about 5 minutes before removing the muffins from the pan; cool on a rack.

Freezer-Friendly Directions: The muffins can be frozen in an airtight container or sealable plastic bag for up to 3 months. Thaw for 3 – 4 hours on the countertop before serving. To reheat, wrap individual muffins in aluminum foil and place in a preheated 350°F oven until warm.

NUTRITION

Serving size:1 muffin
Calories:324
Fat:14 g
Saturated fat:8 g
Carbohydrates:50 g
Sugar:31 g
Fiber:3 g
Protein:5 g
Sodium:293 mg
Cholesterol:52 mg

Dark Chocolate Cake

Prep:30 mins
Cook:30 mins
Additional:20 mins
Servings:12

Ingredients

2 cups boiling water
2 ¾ cups all-purpose flour
2 teaspoons baking soda
½ teaspoon baking powder
1 cup unsweetened cocoa powder
1 cup butter, softened
2 ¼ cups white sugar
½ teaspoon salt
1 ½ teaspoons vanilla extract
4 eggs

Directions

Preheat oven to 350 degrees F. Grease 3 - 9 inch round cake pans. In medium bowl, pour boiling water over cocoa, and whisk until smooth. Let mixture cool. Sift together flour, baking soda, baking powder and salt; set aside.
In a large bowl, cream butter and sugar together until light and fluffy. Beat in eggs one at time, then stir in vanilla. Add the flour mixture alternately with the cocoa mixture. Spread batter evenly between the 3 prepared pans.
Bake in preheated oven for 27 to 30 minutes. Allow to cool.

Nutrition

427 calories; protein 6.6g; carbohydrates 63.5g; fat 18.3g; cholesterol 102.7mg; sodium 462.6mg.

Chocolate Cookies

Servings:12

Ingredients

1 cup packed brown sugar

½ cup shortening

¼ teaspoon baking soda

1 egg

½ cup buttermilk

2 (1 ounce) squares unsweetened chocolate, melted

½ teaspoon salt

1 ½ cups cake flour

1 teaspoon vanilla extract

Directions

Preheat oven to 350 degrees F.

Cream brown sugar, shortening, melted chocolate, egg and buttermilk. Add dry ingredients and beat until smooth.

Drop onto greased cookie sheet and bake for 12 to 15 minutes. Ice with Chocolate Cookie Buttercream Frosting when still warm but not hot.

Spiced Peaches

Prep:20 mins
Cook:50 mins
Additional:12 hrs
Servings:60

Ingredients

6 cups peeled and chopped fresh peaches

3 cups white sugar

½ teaspoon ground allspice

½ teaspoon ground cinnamon

½ teaspoon ground nutmeg

3 tablespoons lemon juice

Directions

Heat five 12-ounce jars in simmering water until ready for use. Wash lids and rings in warm soapy water.

Mix peaches, sugar, lemon juice, cinnamon, nutmeg, and allspice in a large pot. Bring to a boil; cook, stirring occasionally, until peaches are soft, about 15 minutes. Remove from heat.

Mash peaches with an immersion blender or potato masher to desired size and texture. Return to the heat; continue cooking jam until thickened, about 10 minutes more.

Pack jam into hot jars, filling to within 1/4 inch of the top. Wipe rims with a clean, damp cloth. Top with lids and screw on rings.

Place a rack in the bottom of a large stockpot and fill halfway with water. Bring to a boil and lower in jars using a holder, placing them 2 inches apart. Pour in more boiling water to cover the jars by at least 1 inch. Bring the water to a rolling boil, cover the pot, and process for 10 minutes.

Remove the jars from the stockpot and place onto a cloth-covered or wood surface, several inches apart, until cool, about 12 hours. Press the top of each lid with a finger, ensuring that lid does not move up or down and seal is tight.

Nutrition

43 calories; carbohydrates 10.9g; sodium 0.5mg.

Chocolate Pudding Cake

Servings:24

Ingredients

1 (10 inch) angel food cake
1 (8 ounce) container frozen whipped topping, thawed
1 (5.9 ounce) package instant chocolate pudding mix
1 (1.55 ounce) bar milk chocolate

Directions

Tear angel food cake into bite size pieces into a 9x13 inch cake pan (preferably glass).
Prepare chocolate pudding as directed on package. Gently spread over the top of cake pieces, spreading to edges of pan.
Carefully spread whipped topping over chocolate pudding, spreading to edges of pan and taking care not to mix with pudding.
Using a cheese grater or vegetable peeler, grate chocolate bar over the whipped topping.
Chill until ready to serve, at least one hour.

Nutrition

102 calories; protein 1.2g; carbohydrates 17.4g; fat 3.1g; cholesterol 0.4mg; sodium 207mg

Coconut Loaf Cake

Ingredients

The Cake Batter
175 g or ¾ cup softened butter
290 g or 1 ½ cups regular sugar
3 eggs (lightly beaten)
225 g or 1 ¾ cups Plain / All purpose flour (sieved)
175 ml or ¾ cup coconut milk
1 ½ Teaspoons baking powder
6 Tablespoons desiccated / shredded coconut
½ Teaspoon salt

DIRECTIONS

Heat oven to 160c, 300F. Grease and line your baking tin. See here for how to line.

Get all your ingredients ready, i.e coconut, sieve the flour, and add the salt and baking powder to the flour etc.

Start with making the cake batter by creaming the butter and sugar until a pale light color.

Slowly add the beaten eggs to the mixer, on a low-speed setting, a bit at a time. If the mixture starts to curdle or split, add a spoonful of your sieved flour, keep on adding the eggs, and a bit of flour if necessary until all the eggs are added

Add the coconut milk with half of the flour, keeping the mixer on a slow speed. Once combined, add the shredded/desiccated coconut, and the rest of the flour.

Transfer the cake mixture to the greased and lined loaf tin. Then place in the oven for 1 hr and 5 minutes, check after 1 hour.

Have a cup of tea whilst your coconut pound cake is baking and giving off those lovely aromas in your kitchen!

When the cake is done, take it out of the oven and leave in the cake tin until cool. Whilst the cake is still HOT, using a skewer, prick holes all over the top of the cake, pushing the skewer through to the bottom of the cake.

Crab Cakes

Prep:25 mins
Cook:20 mins
Servings:6

Ingredients

⅓ cup dry bread crumbs
¼ red bell pepper, seeded and diced
2 green onions, thinly sliced
¼ green bell pepper, seeded and diced
½ teaspoon hot pepper sauce
1 egg white
2 tablespoons mayonnaise
1 cup canola oil for frying
4 sprigs fresh parsley, chopped
1 tablespoon fresh lemon juice
2 teaspoons Dijon mustard
¼ teaspoon Old Bay TM seasoning
¼ teaspoon dry mustard
½ teaspoon Worcestershire sauce
3 (6 ounce) cans crabmeat, drained and flaked
½ cup dry bread crumbs
¼ teaspoon onion powder

Directions

In a bowl, toss together the 1/3 cup bread crumbs, green bell pepper, red bell pepper, green onions, and parsley. Mix in the egg white, mayonnaise, lemon juice, Worcestershire sauce, and Dijon mustard. Season with Old Bay seasoning, dry mustard, and onion powder. Fold crabmeat into the mixture. Form into 6 large cakes. Coat in the remaining 1/2 cup bread crumbs.

Heat the oil in a large, heavy skillet. Fry the cakes 5 minutes on each side, or until evenly brown. Drain on paper towels.

Nutrition

225 calories; protein 20.7g; carbohydrates 13.8g; fat 9.4g; cholesterol 76.5mg; sodium 508mg

Blackberry Ice Cream

Prep:30 mins
Additional:2 hrs 10 mins
Servings:4

Ingredients

1 pint fresh blackberries
½ teaspoon lemon zest
2 cups heavy cream
½ cup white sugar
1 teaspoon vanilla extract
½ cup whole milk

Directions

Combine blackberries, sugar, and lemon zest in the bowl of a food processor; process until mixture is pureed. Let sit for 10 minutes. Strain the seeds through a fine mesh sieve and return puree to the food processor. Add cream, milk, and vanilla extract. Pulse until mixture is whipped, about 30 seconds.
Pour mixture into an ice cream maker and freeze according to manufacturer's Directions, about 20 minutes. Transfer to an airtight container and freeze until firm, 2 hours to overnight.

Nutrition

560 calories; protein 4.4g; carbohydrates 36.8g; fat 45.4g; cholesterol 166.1mg; sodium 58.3mg.

Tilapia Cakes

Prep:15 mins
Cook:10 mins
Additional:1 hr
Servings:2

Ingredients

2 tablespoons olive oil, divided
2 tilapia fillets
salt and ground black pepper to taste
1 tablespoon dried dill weed
2 green onions, diced
2 tablespoons lemon juice
¼ cup bread crumbs
2 tablespoons crumbled feta cheese
1 tablespoon garlic powder
1 egg
2 teaspoons hot sauce

Directions

Heat a large skillet over medium-high heat. Add 1 tablespoon oil. Add
tilapia fillets, salt, and pepper and cook until easily flaked with a fork,
about 2 minutes on each side. Turn off the heat and shred the fish
with 2 forks. Transfer to a bowl.
Toss the fish with bread crumbs, green onions, egg, lemon juice, feta
cheese, garlic powder, dill, and hot sauce.
Form patties with your hand and refrigerate for at least 1 hour.
Set a skillet over medium-high heat. Add remaining oil. Cook patties in
the hot oil until golden brown, 1 to 3 minutes on each side.

Nutrition

369 calories; protein 30.5g; carbohydrates 15.8g; fat 20.4g; cholesterol 142.3mg; sodium 496.6mg.

Ribbon Cake

Servings:16

Ingredients

1 (8 ounce) package cream cheese

1 egg

½ teaspoon vanilla extract

1 cup all-purpose flour

1 ⅓ cups white sugar

¼ cup white sugar

½ teaspoon vegetable oil

1 ¼ teaspoons baking powder

¼ teaspoon baking soda

1 cup milk

3 tablespoons shortening

½ teaspoon salt

1 egg

3 (1 ounce) squares unsweetened chocolate, melted

3 (1 ounce) squares semisweet chocolate

1 tablespoon butter

½ teaspoon vanilla extract

1 tablespoon water

Directions

In a small bowl, beat together cream cheese, 1/4 cup sugar, 1 egg, and 1/2 teaspoon vanilla until smooth.

In a separate bowl, combine flour, 1 1/3 cup sugar, baking powder, soda, salt, milk, shortening, 1 egg, 1/2 teaspoon vanilla, and 3 squares melted unsweetened chocolate in large mixing bowl. Beat for 1/2 minute with an electric mixer on low speed. Beat 2 minutes on medium speed.

Grease a 9 inch square pan. Pour half of the batter into the pan. Spread cream cheese mixture evenly over the batter, and top with remaining cake batter to cover completely.

Bake at 350 degrees F for 50 to 55 minutes, or until cake tester inserted in center comes out clean. Cool.

Melt 3 squares semisweet chocolate with butter, water, and oil; blend until smooth. Spread evenly over cooled cake.

Nutrition

253 calories; protein 4.2g; carbohydrates 31.6g; fat 13.6g; cholesterol 41.8mg; sodium 193.5mg.

Watermelon Sorbet

Prep:10 mins
Cook:5 mins
Additional:2 hrs 30 mins
Servings:8

Ingredients

1 cup white sugar
3 cups cubed seeded watermelon
¼ cup lemon juice
½ cup water

Directions

Combine sugar, water, and lemon juice in a saucepan over medium
heat; cook and stir until sugar is dissolved, about 5 minutes. Remove
from heat and refrigerate until cooled, about 30 minutes.
Blend watermelon in a blender or food processor until pureed. Stir
pureed watermelon into sugar mixture. Transfer watermelon mixture
to an ice cream maker and freeze according to manufacturer's
Directions.

Nutrition

116 calories; protein 0.4g; carbohydrates 30g; fat 0.1g; sodium 1.1mg.

Hazelnut Cake

Servings:36

Ingredients

1 (18.25 ounce) package devil's food cake mix
1 (3.9 ounce) package instant chocolate pudding mix
¼ cup water
3 cups heavy whipping cream
1 teaspoon vanilla extract
1 cup finely chopped toasted hazelnuts
12 hazelnuts
1 ½ cups semisweet chocolate chips

Directions

Prepare cake mix according to package directions, using required ingredients, plus pudding mix, vanilla, and an additional 1/4 cup of water. Spread batter evenly among three greased and floured 9 inch cake pans. Bake at temperature specified on cake mix box for 18 to 22 minutes, or until a toothpick inserted in the center comes out clean. Let cakes cool completely, then chill in refrigerator for 30 minutes.
In a double boiler over simmering water, melt chocolate chips. Gradually add 1/4 cup of the whipping cream, stirring constantly until smooth. Remove from heat and let cool to room temperature. Beat 3/4 cup of whipping cream until soft peaks form. Fold the whipped cream into the cooled chocolate mixture. Stir in 1/2 cup of the finely chopped hazelnuts. Chill 30 minutes.
Beat remaining 2 cups of whipping cream until soft peaks form, then fold in the remaining 1/2 cup of chopped hazelnuts. Chill until ready to frost cake.
Place 1 cake layer on cake plate. Spread 1/2 of the chilled chocolate mixture over top. Add another cake layer. Spread with other 1/2 of

chocolate mixture. Top with last cake layer. Frost entire cake with hazelnut-whipped cream. Place 12 whole hazelnuts around top outer edge of cake as a garnish. This cake should be kept in the refrigerator.

Nutrition

201 calories; protein 2.5g; carbohydrates 18.4g; fat 13.9g; cholesterol 30mg; sodium 157.3mg.

Pear Muffins

Prep:15 mins
Cook:20 mins
Additional:25 mins
Servings:12

Ingredients

1 cup whole wheat flour

½ cup all-purpose flour

1 ½ teaspoons baking powder

½ teaspoon salt

½ cup low-fat vanilla yogurt

¾ cup white sugar

½ cup canola oil

1 egg

1 ripe pear - peeled, cored, and diced

½ cup chopped pecans

2 teaspoons vanilla extract

Directions

Preheat oven to 450 degrees F. Grease or line 12 muffin cups with
paper liners.

Whisk whole wheat flour, all-purpose flour, sugar, baking powder, and
salt together in a bowl. Whisk yogurt, oil, egg, and vanilla extract
together in a separate bowl until smooth. Stir yogurt mixture into flour
mixture until batter is just mixed; fold in pear and pecans. Spoon
batter into the prepared muffin cups.

Place muffin tin in the preheated oven; reduce heat to 350 degrees F.
Bake until tops of muffins are browned and a toothpick inserted in the
middle comes out clean, 22 to 25 minutes. Cool in the tin for 5
minutes before transferring to a wire rack to cool completely.

Nutrition

240 calories; protein 3.4g; carbohydrates 28.2g; fat 13.4g; cholesterol 16mg; sodium 171.2mg

Spritz Cookies

Servings:24

Ingredients

1 cup butter, softened
1 teaspoon vanilla extract
3 egg yolks
⅔ cup white sugar
2 ½ cups all-purpose flour

Directions

Mix the butter or margarine, sugar, egg yolks and vanilla. Add the flour and mix by hand.
Spoon into cookie press and press onto ungreased cookie sheets.
Sprinkle with colored sugars.
Bake in preheated 400 degrees F oven for 8-10 minutes.

Nutrition

144 calories; protein 1.8g; carbohydrates 15.6g; fat 8.4g; cholesterol 45.9mg; sodium 55.8mg.

Oregano Cookies

yields 2.5 dozen

Ingredients

2 sprigs oregano, about 10 fresh leaves
1 egg
6 oz vegan butter substitute (
6 oz granulated sugar
1 oz (by weight, if you please) good quality molasses
1/2 tsp kosher salt
1/2 tsp baking powder
1 Tbsp fine coffee grounds or 1 tsp freeze-dried instant coffee
7.5 oz all-purpose flour
1/2 tsp baking soda
4 oz 100% Cacao chocolate, chopped fine

Directions

Layer all of the leaves of oregano atop one another and roll into a cigar. Slice quite finely, and then add to the butter. You can melt it together and let it sit, of course, to steep, but if you're in a rush and you just need cookies right now, go ahead and cream it in until it's light and lemon-colored. Add in the sugar and molasses, and cream until quite fluffy, about 2 minutes, scraping down the bowl as needed. Beat in the egg until absolutely emulsified in, about 1 minute, and then scrape down. Remove the bowl from the standing mixer and scrape any butter mixture off the beater with the spatula.

Dump all of the ingredients in, all at once, and stir with a spatula until well-enough combined. Cover with plastic wrap and chill. The cookie does improve when left to rest overnight, but if you can't wait to eat these delicious cookies, just chill the dough in the fridge while the oven heats to 325 degrees F, which should take about 30 minutes. If you can find room in the freezer, even better.

Drop dollops of the cookie dough on to a prepared baking sheet lined with either parchment paper or a silpat mat and bake for 10-12 minutes. If you have a small 1 oz disher, that's ideal. Let the cookies hang out on the sheets for at least 15 minutes before picking them up so they can set. Molasses is an invert sugar, so it's what makes cookies very chewy. In fact, if you're a big fan of chewy cookies, all you have to do to make it super chewy is substitute liquid sugars for granulated/solid ones in some part. I encourage experimentation in all fronts!

If you'd like to make this to be an extra sexy treat, melt some good quality chocolate gently over a double boiler to about body temperature and dip the bottoms of the cookies in, just to coat. Let them harden on parchment paper. You can do that with just about any cookie that you'd like to dress up. You can even straight-up dip half of the cookie and cover it with sprinkles if you're feeling extra festive.

Mango Pudding

Prep:10 mins
Additional:4 hrs
Servings:6

Ingredients

1 cup hot water
2 (.25 ounce) packages powdered gelatin (such as Knox®)
1 cup white sugar
26 ounces canned mango pulp
1 ½ cups evaporated milk
2 (.25 ounce) packages powdered gelatin (such as Knox®)
1 up cold water

Directions

Combine hot water, sugar, and powdered gelatin in a small bowl; stir until sugar and gelatin are dissolved.
Mix mango pulp, evaporated milk, and cold water together in a large bowl. Pour in hot water mixture and stir well.
Refrigerate until set, at least 4 hours.

Nutrition

340 calories; protein 7g; carbohydrates 67.9g; fat 5.1g; cholesterol 18.3mg; sodium 79.9mg.

Carrot Muffins

Servings:24

Ingredients

2 cups all-purpose flour
2 tablespoons baking powder
1 teaspoon salt
2 cups whole wheat flour
1 teaspoon ground cinnamon
¼ teaspoon ground allspice
2 cups finely grated carrots
½ cup packed brown sugar
2 eggs
½ cup molasses
½ cup melted butter
1 cup chopped walnuts
1 cup raisins
2 cups milk

Directions

Preheat oven to 400 degrees F .
Mix wheat and white flours, baking powder, and salt in a large bowl.
Blend in brown sugar, cinnamon, allspice, and grated carrots.
In a mixing bowl beat eggs. Blend in milk, molasses and butter.
Combine this mixture with the flour mixture. Stir until all dry
ingredients are moist.
Spoon mixture into oiled muffin tins adding nuts and raisins if you
would like. Bake for 25 to 35 minutes.

Nutrition

214 calories; protein 4.7g; carbohydrates 32.5g; fat 8.2g; cholesterol 27.3mg; sodium 271.8mg.

Vasilopita

Prep:2 hrs 30 mins
Cook:40 mins
Servings: 8

Ingredients

½ cup warm milk
½ cup bread flour
6 cups bread flour
1 (.25 ounce) package active dry yeast
½ cup white sugar
½ teaspoon ground cinnamon
½ teaspoon ground nutmeg
½ teaspoon salt
¾ cup butter, melted
2 cups warm milk
2 tablespoons butter, melted
1 egg, beaten
1 tablespoon water
3 eggs
½ cup chopped almonds

Directions

In a small bowl, stir together 1/2 cup milk, yeast and 1/2 cup flour. Cover and let the sponge rise in a warm place until nearly doubled in size, about 45 minutes.

Place 6 cups flour in a large bowl. Make a well in the center and add the sponge, salt, sugar, cinnamon, nutmeg, 3/4 cup melted butter, 3 eggs and 2 cups milk. Mix thoroughly to make a stiff dough.

Transfer the dough into a greased springform pan. Brush dough with melted butter, cover with greased plastic wrap, and let rise in a warm place until doubled in size, about 60 to 90 minutes.

Preheat oven to 375 degrees F . Beat egg with 1 tablespoon water to make an egg wash.

When dough has risen, insert a clean silver coin into the loaf. Brush dough egg wash and sprinkle with chopped almonds. Bake in preheated oven until deep golden brown, about 40 minutes.

Nutrition

339 calories; protein 7.5g; carbohydrates 18g; fat 27.2g; cholesterol 152.5mg; sodium 355.2mg.

Coconut Coffee Mousse

Prep:10 mins
Additional:3 hrs 50 mins
Servings:8

Ingredients

1 (8 ounce) container frozen whipped topping, thawed
¼ cup flaked coconut
2 tablespoons coffee flavored liqueur

Directions

Fold coffee liqueur and coconut into whipped topping until well combined. Pour into 8x8 inch baking dish and freeze 4 hours, until firm.

Nutrition

110 calories; protein 0.2g; carbohydrates 8.3g; fat 6.6g; sodium 1.4mg.

Finikia

Prep:45 mins
Cook:25 mins
Servings:60

Ingredients

½ cup butter, softened
1 grated zest of one orange
½ cup corn oil
2 ½ cups all-purpose flour
1 ½ cups semolina
½ cup superfine sugar
1 teaspoon ground cinnamon
1 teaspoon ground cloves
½ cup orange juice
1 cup water
4 teaspoons baking powder
1 cup white sugar
1 cinnamon stick
2 teaspoons lemon juice
½ cup honey
½ cup finely chopped walnuts

Directions

Preheat oven to 350 degrees F . Grease cookie sheets.
In a large bowl, cream together the butter, superfine sugar and orange zest. Gradually mix in the oil and beat until light and fluffy. Combine the flour, semolina, baking powder, cinnamon and cloves; beat into the fluffy mixture alternately with the orange juice. As the mixture thickens, turn out onto a floured board and knead into a firm dough.

Pinch off tablespoonfuls of dough and form them into balls or ovals. Place cookies 2 inches apart onto the prepared cookie sheets.

Bake for 25 minutes in the preheated oven, or until golden. Cool on baking sheets until room temperature.

To make the syrup: In a medium saucepan, over medium heat, combine the water, white sugar, honey, cinnamon stick and lemon juice. Bring to a boil and boil for 10 minutes. Remove the cinnamon stick. While the mixture is boiling hot, dip the cookies in one at a time, making sure to cover them completely. Place them on a wire rack to dry and sprinkle with walnuts. Place paper under the rack to catch the drips. Keep finished cookies in a sealed container at room temperature.

Nutrition

100 calories; protein 1.3g; carbohydrates 14.9g; fat 4.1g; cholesterol 4.1mg; sodium 35.3mg.

Blackberry Cobbler

Prep:20 mins
Cook:25 mins
Servings:8

Ingredients

1 cup all-purpose flour
1 ½ cups white sugar, divided
½ teaspoon salt
6 tablespoons cold butter
1 teaspoon baking powder
2 tablespoons cornstarch
¼ cup cold water
¼ cup boiling water
4 cups fresh blackberries, rinsed and drained
1 tablespoon lemon juice

Directions

Preheat oven to 400 degrees F . Line a baking sheet with aluminum foil.
In a large bowl, mix the flour, 1/2 cup sugar, baking powder, and salt. Cut in butter until the mixture resembles coarse crumbs. Stir in 1/4 cup boiling water just until mixture is evenly moist.
In a separate bowl, dissolve the cornstarch in cold water. Mix in remaining 1 cup sugar, lemon juice, and blackberries. Transfer to a cast iron skillet, and bring to a boil, stirring frequently. Drop dough into the skillet by spoonfuls. Place skillet on the foil lined baking sheet. Bake 25 minutes in the preheated oven, until dough is golden brown.

Baked Plums

Prep:10 mins
Cook:40 mins
Servings:12

Ingredients

½ cup butter
5 eggs
1 cup dried currants
1 cup golden raisins
¾ cup white sugar
1 tablespoon all-purpose flour
3 cups bread cubes
2 teaspoons ground cinnamon
½ teaspoon ground allspice
½ cup chopped pecans
½ teaspoon pumpkin pie spice
½ teaspoon ground cloves

Directions

Preheat oven to 350 degrees F .
Cream together butter and sugar. Beat in eggs, one at a time, until fully incorporated. In a separate bowl, toss currants, raisins and pecans with flour. Fold into butter mixture. Fold in bread, cinnamon, allspice, cloves and pumpkin pie spice. Pour into an 8x8 inch baking dish.
Bake in preheated oven 40 minutes, until set.

Nutrition

265 calories; protein 4.6g; carbohydrates 34.5g; fat 13.4g; cholesterol 97.8mg; sodium 145.5mg.

Yogurt Cookies

Prep:10 mins
Cook:12 mins
Servings:36

Ingredients

½ cup packed brown sugar
½ cup white sugar
½ cup plain nonfat yogurt
¼ cup margarine or butter
¼ cup shortening
2 teaspoons vanilla extract
1 ¾ cups all-purpose flour
½ teaspoon salt
2 cups semisweet chocolate chips
½ teaspoon baking soda

Directions

Preheat the oven to 375 degrees F. Grease cookie sheets.
In a medium bowl, cream together the brown sugar, white sugar, margarine and shortening until light and fluffy. Stir in yogurt and vanilla. Combine the flour, baking soda, and salt; stir into the creamed mixture until incorporated, then mix in chocolate chips. Drop by rounded teaspoonfuls 2 inches apart onto the prepared cookie sheets. Bake for 8 to 10 minutes in the preheated oven, until the edges begin to brown. Cool for a minute on the cookie sheets before removing to wire racks to cool completely.

Nutrition

115 calories; protein 1.2g; carbohydrates 16.6g; fat 5.5g; cholesterol 0.1mg; sodium 68.3mg.

Galaktoboureko

Prep:1 hr
Cook:45 mins
Servings:15

Ingredients

1 cup semolina flour
3 ½ tablespoons cornstarch
1 cup white sugar
6 cups whole milk
¼ teaspoon salt
½ cup white sugar
1 teaspoon vanilla extract
12 sheets phyllo dough
6 eggs
1 cup water
1 cup white sugar
¾ cup butter, melted

Directions

Pour milk into a large saucepan, and bring to a boil over medium heat. In a medium bowl, whisk together the semolina, cornstarch, 1 cup sugar and salt so there are no cornstarch clumps. When milk comes to a boil, gradually add the semolina mixture, stirring constantly with a wooden spoon. Cook, stirring constantly until the mixture thickens and comes to a full boil. Remove from heat, and set aside. Keep warm. In a large bowl, beat eggs with an electric mixer at high speed. Add 1/2 cup of sugar, and whip until thick and pale, about 10 minutes. Stir in vanilla.
Fold the whipped eggs into the hot semolina mixture. Partially cover the pan, and set aside to cool.

Preheat the oven to 350 degrees F.

Butter a 9x13 inch baking dish, and layer 7 sheets of phyllo into the pan, brushing each one with butter as you lay it in. Pour the custard into the pan over the phyllo, and cover with the remaining 5 sheets of phyllo, brushing each sheet with butter as you lay it down.

Bake for 40 to 45 minutes in the preheated oven, until the top crust is crisp and the custard filling has set. In a small saucepan, stir together the remaining cup of sugar and water. Bring to a boil. When the Galaktoboureko comes out of the oven, spoon the hot sugar syrup over the top, particularly the edges. Cool completely before cutting and serving. Store in the refrigerator.

Nutrition

391 calories; protein 8.3g; carbohydrates 55.7g; fat 15.4g; cholesterol 108.6mg; sodium 244.9mg.

Vanilla Meringue

Prep:20 mins
Cook:1 hr 30 mins
Additional:1 hr 30 mins
Servings:12

Ingredients

2 egg whites
½ cup white sugar
½ vanilla bean
1 tablespoon vanilla extract
⅛ teaspoon cream of tartar

Directions

Preheat the oven to 225 degrees F. Line a large baking sheet with parchment paper.

Place egg whites and cream of tartar into a large bowl; beat using an electric mixer at medium speed until soft peaks form. Increase speed to high and add sugar 1 tablespoon at a time while mixing until stiff peaks form. Scrape seeds from vanilla bean into the bowl and add vanilla extract; beat just until blended.

Spoon batter into a pastry bag and pipe mounds onto the prepared baking sheet.

Bake in the preheated oven until set, about 1 1/2 hours. Turn oven off; let cookies cool in the closed oven for 1 1/2 hours. Remove cookies carefully from paper.

Nutrition

40 calories; protein 0.6g; carbohydrates 9.1g; sodium 9.4mg.

Pumpkin Ice Cream

Prep:15 mins
Cook:15 mins
Additional:3 hrs
Servings:8

Ingredients

1 ½ cups half-and-half
¾ cup white sugar
½ teaspoon vanilla extract
1 ½ cups canned pumpkin
¾ teaspoon pumpkin pie spice
6 egg yolks
1 ½ cups heavy whipping cream

Directions

Heat half-and-half in a saucepan over medium-low heat to just below a boil, about 5 minutes.

Beat egg yolks, sugar, and vanilla extract together in a bowl using a whisk until smooth. Gradually pour half-and-half into egg mixture to temper the eggs; add pumpkin pie spice.

Pour the half-and-half mixture back into the saucepan; cook and stir over medium-low heat to just before boiling until mixture thickens, about 10 minutes. Remove saucepan from heat and beat pumpkin and whipping cream into half-and-half mixture until smooth; strain through a fine-mesh strainer into a bowl. Refrigerate pumpkin mixture until completely chilled, at least 1 hour.

Transfer pumpkin mixture to an ice cream maker and follow manufacturers' Directions for making ice cream.

Nutrition

342 calories; protein 4.7g; carbohydrates 26.3g; fat 25.2g; cholesterol 231.6mg; sodium 152.4mg.

CHAPTER 6: SMOOTHIES AND DRINKS

Almonds and Zucchini Smoothie

Prep Time: 5 mins
Total Time: 5 mins

Ingredients

12 oz. unsweetened almond milk
1–2 scoop vanilla protein powder
1/2 cup frozen blueberries
1 TBS roasted almond butter
1 TBS ground chia seed
1 cup steamed and frozen green zucchini (or sub frozen caulilflower)

Directions

Ensure that you have steamed and frozen zucchini on hand or make it at least 8 hours in advance before starting recipe
Add all ingredients to high speed blender and process until smooth and creamy. Add more almond milk to reach thinner consistency and a little more blueberries or zucchini for thicker consistency. Pour into a large mason jar and enjoy topped with fresh blueberries, almond butter, and ground chia seeds.

Banana Apple Smoothie

Prep:5 mins
Servings:2

Ingredients

1 frozen bananas, peeled and chopped
1 Gala apple, peeled, cored and chopped
½ cup orange juice
¼ cup milk

Directions

In a blender combine frozen banana, orange juice, apple and milk. Blend until smooth. pour into glasses and serve.

Nutrition

132 calories; protein 2.3g; carbohydrates 30.9g; fat 1g; cholesterol 2.4mg; sodium 14.4mg.

Avocado with Walnut Butter Smoothie

Total Time5 Mins
Serves2

INGREDIENTS

1 cup low fat milk (or substitute non-dairy milk of choice)
2 tablespoons California Walnuts
1 frozen banana
1 teaspoon matcha powder
12 fresh mint leaves
1 tablespoon lime juice
2 ice cubes
1/4 avocado
1 tablespoon honey

Directions

Place all ingredients in a high-speed blender and blend until smooth.

Lime Spinach Smoothie

Prep:20 mins
Total:20 mins
Servings:3

Ingredients

1 large cucumber, chopped
1 lime, juiced
2 apples, cored and chopped
½ cup cold water, or more as needed
2 cups fresh spinach
1 bunch fresh parsley
1 (1 inch) piece fresh ginger, peeled and chopped
3 ribs celery, chopped
½ lemon, juiced

Directions

Place cucumber, apples, celery, water, spinach, parsley, ginger, lime juice, and lemon juice in a blender; blend until smooth.

Nutrition

89 calories; protein 2.5g; carbohydrates 21.4g; fat 0.6g; sodium 82.7mg.

Caramel Latte

Ingredients

3 fluid ounces brewed espresso
1 tablespoon caramel sauce
2 tablespoons whipped cream
¾ cup milk
½ cups ice cubes
2 tablespoons white sugar

Directions

Place the espresso, caramel sauce, and sugar into a blender pitcher. Blend on high until the caramel and sugar dissolve into the espresso. Pour in the milk and add the ice; continue blending until smooth and frothy. Top with whipped cream to serve.

Nutrition

293 calories; protein 6.8g; carbohydrates 47.5g; fat 9.3g; cholesterol 35.4mg; sodium 164.1mg.

Dandelion Tea

PREP TIME 5 mins
COOK TIME 20 mins
TOTAL TIME 25 mins...
SERVINGS 4 cups...

INGREDIENTS

2 cup dandelion all parts
4 cups water boiled

DIRECTIONS

Clean dandelion
Boil water Pour boiling water over dandelion
Cover water and dandelions with a lid...

Lemon Pina Colada

YIELDMakes 2 servings

INGREDIENTS

1/2 cup canned sweetened cream of coconut (such as Coco López)
6 tablespoons citrus-flavored rum
1/4 cup chilled whipping cream
6 tablespoons white rum
3 tablespoons fresh lemon juice
Grated lemon peel
Ground nutmeg
4 cups crushed ice
3/4 cup pineapple juice

Directions

Place first 6 ingredients in large blender. Add ice. Cover and blend until smooth. Pour into two 14-ounce glasses. Garnish with grated lemon peel and nutmeg.
Coconut Rim
Dip the rim of each glass in water, then press into a bowl of coarsely crushed toasted shredded coconut. To crush the coconut easily, rub it several times in the palm of your hand.

Herbal Tea

Prep:5 mins
Cook:2 mins
Servings:4

Ingredients

1 quart water, or as needed
1 teaspoon ground cumin
1 teaspoon grated fresh ginger
1 tablespoon honey
1 teaspoon lime juice
3 leaves fresh mint
1 teaspoon grated lime zest

Directions

Bring water to a boil in a pot; stir in honey, cumin, ginger, lime zest, lime juice, and mint. Cook and stir until flavors are infused, about 2 minutes.

Nutrition

19 calories; protein 0.1g; carbohydrates 4.8g; fat 0.1g; sodium 8.3mg.

Cranberry-Hazelnut Coffee Cake

Prep:20 mins
Cook:1 hr 15 minsServings:
12

Ingredients

1 ¾ cups cake flour
1 teaspoon baking powder
 teaspoon salt
¾ cup unsalted butter
1 teaspoon baking soda
4 eggs
2 ½ teaspoons vanilla extract
1 teaspoon ground cinnamon
¾ cup whole milk
1 ½ cups dark brown sugar
¼ cup dried cranberries
¼ cup chopped toasted hazelnuts
¼ cup white sugar
1 teaspoon ground cinnamon
⅓ cup dark brown sugar

Directions

Preheat oven to 350 degrees F. Butter and flour a 9 inch springform
pan. Sift together the flour, baking powder, baking soda and salt; set
aside.
In a large bowl, cream together the butter and 1 1/2 cup sugar until
light and fluffy. Beat in the eggs one at a time, then stir in the vanilla
and 1 teaspoon cinnamon. Beat in the flour mixture alternately with
the milk. Fold in cranberries and hazelnuts. Pour batter into prepared

pan. Mix together 1/3 cup brown sugar, 1/4 cup white sugar, and 1 teaspoon cinnamon; sprinkle over cake, and swirl through the batter. Bake in the preheated oven for 75 to 80 minutes, or until a toothpick inserted into the center of the cake comes out clean. Allow to cool.

Nutrition

380 calories; protein 4.8g; carbohydrates 57.2g; fat 15.3g; cholesterol 94mg; sodium 283.3mg.

Sherbet Shake

READY IN: 10mins
SERVES: 4

INGREDIENTS

1quart sherbet, any flavor (I use rainbow flavor)
1/2liter carbonated carbonated lemon-lime beverage (7 Up is the best)

DIRECTIONS

Mix 1/2 quart of sherbet & 1/4 liter of soda together in a blender.
Repeat with the other half of the ingredients.
Serve chilled in a glass.

Cinnamon Apple Water

Ingredients:

One gallon water (filtered or bottled)
6 Cinnamon Sticks
5-6 Apples

Directions

Bring water to boil and then reduce to low heat to simmer.
Core and slice your apples – This handy tool – apple corer and slicer may help.
Try to slice apples as thin as possible!
Add apples and cinnamon sticks to your simmering water.
Simmer 45 minutes. Let stand and cool.
Strain water into glass pitcher.
Enjoy fresh right away.
You may enjoy it at room temperature or refrigerate for up to 5 days.
You may discard the cooked apples or eat them for a gut health

Nectarin Juice

Prep:5 mins
Cook:0 mins
Total:5 mins

Ingredients

2 Nectarines
1-2 tablespoons of your favorite seeds or nuts such
as Pumpkin, Walnut, Sesame or Almond
For a wonderful smoothie add 1-2 cups of Oat, Rice, Almond or cow's
milk
3-4 leaves of your favorite green such as Kale, Spinach or my
favorite, Wheatgrass
2 Carrots

Directions

Gather the ingredients.
Blend.
Note that there are no added sweeteners even in this smoothie recipe.
This is because the recipe is delicious without added sugar.

CPSIA information can be obtained
at www.ICGtesting.com
Printed in the USA
BVHW012113260321
603406BV00017B/83

9 781802 237030